Eat
FOR THE
Health
of It

MARTHA A. ERICKSON
with Barbara L. Dempsey

Eat
FOR THE
Health
of It

MARTHA A. ERICKSON
with Barbara L. Dempsey

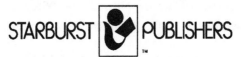

STARBURST PUBLISHERS

P. O. Box 4123, Lancaster, Pennsylvania 17604

To schedule Author appearances write:
Author Appearances, Starburst Promotions, P.O. Box 4123,
Lancaster, Pennsylvania 17604 or call (717) 293-0939

Credits:
Cover art by Terry Dugan Design

Eat for the Health of It

First Printing, June, 1997

ISBN: 0-914984-78-0
Library of Congress Catalog Number 96-068836
Printed in the United States of America

COMMENTS

"Martha Erickson has written a well researched book about health and nutrition."
Ara Parseghian, Chairman, Ara Parseghian Medical Research Foundation, and former Notre Dame head football coach

"*Eat For The Health Of It* is a rare opportunity to see how an expert in the field of clinical nutrition provides the vital link between medical care and individual nutrition requirements."
Anna Uhran, R.D.

"I thank the Lord every day for sending me to you. I really appreciate what you did for my health and my peace of mind. Thank you very much!"
Marietta Frick (former patient)

"In *Eat For The Health Of It* Martha Erickson reveals the true facts about nutrition and how you too can improve your health."
Margaret B. Salmon, R.D., Author and President Salmon Consultants, Nutritionists

"By sharing her knowledge, wisdom and insights, Martha Erickson is making a lasting contribution to the health of America."
Arthur J. Decio, CEO, Skyline Corporation

ACKNOWLEDGMENTS

I Wish to thank my husband, G. Walter Erickson, M.D., South Bend Clinic, South Bend, Indiana for his patience, guidance and medical knowledge.

Carol W. Erickson, Journalism and English teacher, Garwood.

E. Erickson, Vice President, Great Lakes Technologies Group, Royal Oak, Michigan, and Christopher L. Erickson, computer expert, for their wealth of knowledge in the computer and journalism fields.

Quincy Erickson, member of the Women Chefs of America and Director of Schlotzsky's Brands Inc., Austin, Texas, for her superb knowledge of food and the food industry.

Virginia and William Anzelc, Vice President and President respectively, Anjon Nutrition Analysis Systems, South Bend, Indiana.

Don McLane, engineer and computer professional, Mishawaka, Indiana.

My patients who inspired me to write this book.

Barbara L. Dempsey and I dedicate *Eat for the Health of It* to the members of our families. May they live long, happy and healthy lives.

IMPORTANT NOTICE

TABLE OF CONTENTS

INTRODUCTION

WHAT happens when the body, which depends on food for fuel, runs out of incoming nutrients and calories or is unable to process certain foods? Unlike a car which stops when it runs out of gasoline, or a piece of machinery that breaks down when it is not maintained, body parts never go on vacation. The heart continues to beat, the blood to flow, the brain to think, the lungs to breathe—even without fuel from food.

Most of us never worry about what happens until we get sick or do not have enough energy. Vaguely we think our body will take care of itself. We think we can make up for a skipped meal at another meal. We think we can eat vitamin and mineral supplements instead of eating food. We think that if we get sick we can let our doctors fix us up. We think we know how to feed ourselves—eat a low-fat diet, take vitamins, exercise and don't eat too much.

There is a common belief that the less you eat the more body fat you will lose, the more calories you consume the more weight you will gain. That belief is too simple, a summary of a very complex subject and is wrought with pitfalls, one of which is how people interpret it.

You know you can eat too much food, but did you know you can eat too little? Has anyone warned you of the consequences of following a low fat diet?

The strongest factor which controls your body and your future health is what you choose to eat and when. This book explains what happens and suggests some solutions to help you control sleeplessness, high blood cholesterol, headaches, intestinal problems, hypoglycemia, diabetes and difficulty in breathing.

The theme of *Eat for the Health of It* is very fundamental: feed your operating system, not your body fat, and thus protect your health. When you lose cells from your operating system, you can lose your health. Every single minute that you are alive, it is your operating system (lean tissue) which continually uses calories and nutrients. Body fat uses virtually none. Therefore, your first need is to calculate your daily caloric needs. Since each person has a different amount of lean tissue, each has a different caloric need. This book shows you how to calculate your need.

Of course, when you consume more calories than your operating system can use, the extra calories are deposited as a coat of fat, hindering the body's operation. You may develop health problems. Even if you eat less calories to lose the body fat, you still must eat enough to support your operating system.

The focus of your health then moves from just losing weight to saving your operating system. It changes the way you take care of yourself. Although this book is not a weight loss book, I have learned that when health returns often body fat is lost.

Ralph Waldo Emerson said, "The first wealth is health." Millions of Americans are spending their wealth trying to find health when it is right here under their noses. Eating in a healthy way is the basic concept for preserving and restoring health.

Preserving health is not as profitable as treating an illness. In addition, solving nutritional problems is complicated, given the lifestyles of people and given the various environments people live in. People want simple answers to complex problems. Their demand has spawned an enormously profitable industry—an industry that promotes medications and drugs, supplements, powders and chemicals. As a way to prevent and treat diseases and disorders, adequate nutrition has no equal at saving health care costs and lives.

This book is not a substitute for appropriate medical treatment. It can supply some facts about food and nutrition which can enhance medical treatment, as it did for many people in my practice. Case histories illustrate how patients were able to bring a variety of major and minor diseases under their control with the food they needed to protect and repair their bodies. As an example, you can learn how adequate calories and nutrients helped a woman with Ehler-Danlos syndrome recover her muscles, how a man reduced his blood cholesterol in 10 days without medication and how a woman who had diarrhea for 25 years was able to travel without worrying about the next bathroom.

This book uses no gimmicks, applies no controversial methods. It follows the precepts and recommendations from the United States Surgeon General's office, the American Diabetes Association, The American Cancer Society, The American Heart Association,

The American Dietetic Association and the American Medical Association. Their recommendations of small amounts of protein and fat and large amounts of carbohydrates are best presented visually with the pyramid of the food groups. The book uses these recommendations to demonstrate why the pyramid works and why people become healthier.

Eat for the Health of It will change the way you think about meals, food and their connection to your health. If you follow the clear guidelines you may be able to restore and maintain your own health or the health of loved ones.

As a Registered Dietitian in private practice and as a college instructor for the past 15 years, I have counseled many patients and taught college students how to protect their operating systems by consuming enough calories and nutrients on a regular basis. Because no two individuals are alike and because many individual have various nutritional problems and complications, I relied on contemporary and historical medical and nutritional research for help. The results have been exciting. Some of these cases are illustrated in the book to show how the research was used.

The road to nutritional health is not a freeway for many people. But once you experience how smoothly your body machinery can run, you can become motivated and learn new habits. The road may be long, rough, and full of obstacles. So what if you stumble? You are learning some basic rules to maintain your health—to understand the signals from your body, what to do about them and to *Eat for the Health of It.*

How to Use This Book

The book is organized into chapters with sub headings. Within the paragraphs, you will find references to chapter notes. The notes contain more technical, in depth and/or "how to" information. Further information about a subject mentioned in the book can be obtained by reading the articles that are cited as references and in the bibliography. The appendix has further information about resources.

CHAPTER 1

The Body Never Goes On Vacation
But You May Pay For One Anyway

MOST people assume that if they don't eat, the fat on their bodies will be used for energy. What people have heard for decades is that the more calories they eat, the more weight they will gain; the less they eat the more weight they will lose. What kind of weight do they mean—body fat or lean tissue weight? It makes a big difference as far as health is concerned.

What really happens in our bodies and how we can use this information to preserve or recover our health is the subject of this book.

The body is comprised of two sets of cells—lean tissue and fat. Most people seem to know that muscles are lean body mass and that they use energy. Covert Bailey first said in his book, *Fit or Fat,*[1] that the body's active metabolizing tissue, muscle, not fat, determines the number of calories needed each day. His rationale was that the more one exercises, the more muscle tissue one builds, the more one can eat. This is true.

Basic Caloric Needs

But there is more to the metabolizing tissue than muscle. It includes all the other working parts: brain, nerves, heart, lungs, stomach, intestines, skin, bones, blood, immune system, hormones, enzymes, the liver, kidney, bladder, ovaries, uterus, urinary tract, etc. These parts use calories too. Fat cells use very few. Fat is passive tissue.

In the past, to determine a person's daily caloric needs, total weight was used as the yardstick. This equation was not questioned, despite the fact that if a person weighed 400 pounds, he or she would need 3800 calories a day. When body fat is removed from the equation and lean tissue is determined, this same 400 pound person needs only 2500 calories a day. An overweight person is simply a lean person coated with extra fat. Therefore, the number of calories each of us needs daily to maintain our health status is based on the number of our lean cells. *And each of us has a different amount.*

To understand the difference, we can compare the body to a car. A Volkswagen needs less fuel than a Mack truck because its parts are smaller and it weighs less. It is similar to the human body. The amount of fuel that we need each day depends on the sum of our *lean* parts. Let us use as examples a woman named Robin, and a man named Gary. Both have the same amount of body fat. Robin is 5'5" tall and weighs 130 pounds. She needs less fuel than Gary who is 6'1" tall and weighs 170 pounds. The difference is in the size of their *operating systems.* Robin has smaller bones, less muscle, smaller organs and less skin than Gary.

The sum of our lean tissue cells can be determined by four common methods. Exercise physiologists, Katch, Katch and McArdle describe them in their book, *Exercise Physiology.*[2] Of the four, I prefer to use the circumference measurement tables. Measuring with a measuring tape is easy and uncomplicated, especially when I want to monitor a person's lean tissue and body fat weekly. With this method, three measurements are taken. One is the waist measurement where fat increases or decreases in size.

Using the circumference measurement tables, Robin has 120 pounds of lean tissue and Gary has 145 pounds. To calculate their base caloric needs, we can apply a little known formula (described in chapter notes) to calculate their base calories. Robin needs 2000 calories and Gary needs 2400 calories. Generally, women need a base of 2000 to 2400 calories whereas men need 2400 to 3000 calories. A base number does not factor in calories for aerobic exercise, illness, age, environmental temperature and body insulation. Calculating calories for anyone is somewhat imprecise. Although this method is not perfect, it produces numbers for individuals that are fairly accurate and is flexible enough to add calories for other factors.

The base calories support the lean tissue which is made up of various parts of the body. Each part of the body has been assigned an approximate amount of calories it may use.

The *brain* and *nerves*: *600* calories. The *brain* has a higher priority for calories than muscles or any other part. It is like a conductor of a symphony orchestra who coordinates what the cells do and how they react to each other. Nothing can work in the body without direction from the brain. The *nerves* carry the signals from the brain to the rest of the body. These two, the brain and nerves, use more energy than any other organ. Other parts of the body must compete for the remaining fuel.

The *heart* and *lungs: 300* calories. *The heart* muscle beats about 110,000 times a day and *the lungs* breathe in and out 18 times a minute.

The *stomach* and *intestinal tract: 200 to 300* calories (10 percent of the total calories). The peristaltic muscles carry food through 26 feet of the *intestinal tract*. Enzymes are produced here and digest the food into single molecules.

The *liver* and *blood* system: *300 to 400* calories. The *liver* processes chemicals, makes cholesterol, and produces blood glucose, the body's main fuel supply. The *blood* carries the nutrients and glucose to every cell. Muscles in the blood vessels move the blood along its 60,000 mile route in 80 seconds.

The *bones* and *muscles: 500 to 800* calories. This many calories are needed to move the weight around and to hold the body erect but these calories do not factor in exercise. Bones need energy to store and release materials for the body. Everything in the body weighs something. For instance our head and liver are four percent of the body's weight whereas muscles are 35 to 40 percent and fat may weigh as much as 55 percent. A large boned person starts with more weight to carry around than a small boned person.

Miscellaneous parts: *100* calories. To name a few: *Eyes* see. *Ears* hear. *Hormones* and *enzyme* systems react and try to keep the body in balance. The *immune system* fends off bacteria, viruses and allergies. It can be compared to a trillion firemen fighting millions of fires, all day long, 365 days a year.

More or Less Calories

After the basic number of calories is determined, calories must be added or subtracted for other factors. These other factors are body insulation, exercise, environmental temperature, and illness.

Body Insulation: With less insulation or body fat, more calories are needed to maintain the body at 98.6 degrees Fahrenheit. Vital organs do not perform at their peak in a body that is too cool or too hot (as with a fever). The body can be compared to a house. Both have furnaces that require fuel. The body house needs food for fuel too. Less insulation in a house means more fuel is needed to keep it warm. The same with the body house. Less fat insulation means it needs more fuel. For each percent below the normal percent body fat, I add 100 calories. For adult women, normal body fat is 18 percent, whereas for adult men it is 20 percent, (using the circumference measurement). Children have different criteria for percentage of normal body fat. Other measuring devices have their own standards for body fat.

I didn't realize the importance of body insulation until a woman brought her teenage son to consult with me. He had only two percent body fat. He had little energy and was unable to concentrate in school. This 14-year-old's body temperature was 97 degrees. His mother said he was too tired to get up for breakfast and he regularly skipped lunch. By adding 1600 calories to his base number, a total of 3000 calories daily was needed for his body to function properly. With his mother's help, he was encouraged to eat 1,000 calories each meal for one week to see if it made any difference.

He followed the meal plan and reported back the next week. I thought he would report that he performed better in school, slept better at night, ran faster in his track events, was less irritable, felt better or had more energy overall. Instead he reported he was *warmer*. His body temperature had risen to 98.6 F.

Before starting the 3000 calorie diet, this young man was dragging and listless. He had sallow skin. His eyes and hair were dull. At his track meet six weeks later, his hair was platinum blond and shone, his blue eyes sparkled, his complexion was clear and he had lots of energy. And he won the race.

Calories are next added for aerobic exercise or strenuous work which require more oxygen. For each hour of aerobic exercise, the body demands 300-500 more calories. During aerobic exercise, walking, bicycling, swimming, dancing, running, cross country skiing and skating, the legs and arms do the work and the body is forced to inhale more oxygen.

Conversely, in aerobic exercise, the body expends more oxygen, using less calories. When I calculate calories, I do not add calories for lifting weights, floor exercises, calisthenics, housework, or carrying a child around.

However, I do add an additional 300 to 500 calories for each hour of strenuous work such as ditch-digging, truck-loading, heavy construction, or farming. The total may be as much as 6000 calories.

A *growing* child needs an extra 500 calories a day. A *pregnant* woman needs an extra 300 calories a day for her growing fetus. The growing child and the fetus each are adding 200,000 cells a minute! At the other end of the lifeline, as the body ages, many lean tissue cells have been lost through the years, so the body will need less calories. But it may need the calories more often through the day. How many calories are needed is determined by measuring for lean tissue.

Weather is another consideration when determining calories. Like a family house, the body house usually needs more furl in winter than in summer. Athletes with only two-to-four percent body fat or women who have less than 14 percent may have more difficulty maintaining normal body temperature in the winter unless they eat more, add layers of clothing, or turn up the thermostat in the house. In summer, when the outside temperature approaches or exceeds body temperature, additional calories are needed to cool the body. These caloric needs change slightly from day to day.

Calories need to be added for illness or injury, both of which force the body to demand more calories. It is lean tissue, not body fat, that works harder to fight off germs, bacteria, and viruses and to repair itself. For example, a person who is severely burned needs 4000 to 6000 calories a day to aid in repairing skin and tissue.

The total calories that we may need each day, then, depends on our lean body mass (lean tissue), body fat (insulation), physical activity, age, environmental temperature and illness.

Of course there are people who consume more calories than their lean cells can use and others who consume too few. In the past, people could not tell from the weight on the scale whether they gained or lost body fat or lean tissue. But, there *is* a way and that is using measurement. For example, let's consider a woman whose body fat is 15 percent. Once her calories are calculated, using the formula based on her lean tissue, an extra 300 calories a day must be added because she has three percent insulation below the base of 18 percent body fat. If she exercises an hour a day, she needs to add another 300 calories. Therefore, she will need to add 600 calories to a base of 2000 for a total of 2600 calories. If she had not been eating this many calories she would have retained more body fat and lost lean tissue. But it is lean tissue weight, not fat, that determines caloric need.

Here's another example. A woman has 24 percent body fat and, based on her lean tissue weight, her caloric need is 2400. To lose body fat, *her first consideration must be to protect her lean tissue cells*. Therefore, she can only subtract 300 to 500 calories from the base of 2400 calories. And she must exercise to burn off anymore calories. Diet alone will not help her lose body fat, because a diet too low in calories will result in the loss of lean tissue pounds too.

Men are no different from women. They must protect their lean tissue cells. To lose body fat, they can subtract 300 to 500 calories from a base of say 2700, but they must exercise away another 300 to 500 calories daily.

Monitoring Health Status

Measuring people for body fat and lean tissue has a critically important advantage. It can actually be used to evaluate and track a person's health status. If lean tissue is lost, health is being lost. The focus of a person's health moves from losing weight to saving lean tissue. It changes the way people take care of themselves. Feed your lean tissue and save your health. And very often when health returns, body fat is lost. This may seem too simple at first glance . . . but it works.

I first realized the usefulness of this system when I was fortunate to monitor a woman who had Diabetes Type II. Even though she was consuming 1800 calories a day, she lost 53 pounds of which 48 was body fat. I could detect the difference when I measured and weighed her. The results were what we had hoped. Her blood pressure and blood cholesterol levels dropped to normal, her energy level increased and her diabetic symptoms disappeared. Her health returned and she lost body fat.

Another woman whom I monitored for a year, developed a cold on three separate occasions. With each cold, she lost about five pounds of lean tissue cells and gained about three to four pounds of body fat cells! But then the numbers reversed themselves when the woman recovered. This further convinced me that measuring people for lean body mass and body fat was an important benchmark by which to evaluate and track a person's physical wellness.

The Body Without Energy From Food

Yes, it is important that people do not skip meals and consume enough calories and nutrients to support their lean tissue cells. But why? The body parts will continue to work for days without food. The heart still beats, lungs still breathe, ears continue to hear, eyes see, throats swallow, limbs move. If the body were a car it would stop. But I'm talking about the human body which continues to live and the parts continue to work. Where does the energy come from, body fat? Don't we wish!

The energy comes from glucose. Every cell in the body must have glucose. Glucose comes from only two sources: food or lean tissue. Fat can never be converted to glucose except when the body is in a starvation state. The best and most efficient source of glucose from food is starch carbohydrates. One hundred percent is converted to glucose. Whereas, with lean tissue and dietary protein only 50 percent can be converted to glucose. Not only is lean tissue an inefficient source of glucose, it leaves undesirable waste products that must be excreted. Although some cells can use blood fats for energy, the brain, nerves, and red blood cells cannot. They use glucose exclusively and take priority for it above all other cells. Additionally, even the cells that use fat must have glucose to convert it to energy.

Glucose is delivered to the cells by the blood. Perhaps you have had a blood test to determine the glucose level. The amount of glucose in the blood is controlled by the liver and several hormones. Starch carbohydrates are digested in the intestinal tract to glucose and travel to the liver where, if there is enough, the glucose can be stored in the liver and muscles as glycogen. The glycogen is then converted back to glucose as it is needed by the cells. But if there is not enough starch carbohydrates in the meals, glycogen is not stored.

When people follow a low-calorie diet or fast, they may not consume enough starch carbohydrates. By the end of the first day, the liver has run out of glycogen. It must find another source of glucose. So it extracts 90 percent from the protein in lean tissue cells and ten percent from body fat. The loss of protein means the loss of the cell. If the loss of these lean tissue cells were to continue, the person would die when 25 to 30 percent is gone. That would take about three weeks—even if the person was obese. However, the body does not allow that to happen. On the third day, the thyroid hormone signals the cells to slow down and also signals the liver to increase its breakdown of body fat. Waste products from this breakdown are acids. Lean tissue yields uric *acid* and body fat yields huge quantities (90 to 95 percent) of fatty *acids*. The blood becomes even more *acidic* with the loss of potassium, sodium and water, the very elements that would neutralize the acidity. Plain and simple, *acid* blood or ketosis develops.

Ketosis indicates that the liver is laboring to produce glucose to satisfy cell demand. With protein yielding only 50 percent glucose and fat even less . . . 5 to 10 percent, the conversion to glucose is too slow and the amount too small to allow the liver to meet the body's glucose demands. The body comes under stress.

Ketosis can develop when food intake is inadequate either by choice or from illness. Many diet programs promote ketosis as a "harmless" way for people to burn fat and to lose weight. Yes, weight is lost, but not without a price. Most people assume they are losing body fat. Actually, when they are measured, of the ten pounds they may lose, four pounds will be fat but six pounds will be water (which contains vital nutrients) and lean tissue.

People who are trying to lose weight are so delighted to see the loss of pounds, they may ignore the signs and symptoms of lost lean tissue cells and continue on their restrictive ketosis diet. The symptoms are dehydration, rashes, and/or erratic heartbeat, headaches, lack of appetite and energy, dizziness, weakness, and cramping. Many individuals may have been told that these symptoms are a necessary part of losing weight. They are not. They signal a dangerous condition. Any time lean tissue is lost, health is at risk.

Can Organs Shrink?

As the number of lean tissue cells are converted to glucose, the organs shrink. Fewer cells in the organs are left to do the jobs. Many cells do not return. Without 100 percent of the cells available to work, and less "workers," the vital organs must adapt to the lower number of incoming calories by slowing down. Body fat is conserved. The body conserves calories by lowering its thermostat, because maintaining a temperature of 98.6 degrees is not a priority. We may do the same thing in our houses when we want to conserve energy. We lower the thermostat. One difference is this: in our houses, we voluntarily lower the temperature. In our bodies, the temperature is involuntarily reduced when there isn't enough fuel to go around. Body temperature can be a measure of illness and the loss of lean tissue.

Losing lean tissue cells can happen to you or to anyone on any day. Just skipping meals results in the loss of lean tissue cells. As the title of this chapter states, the body is never on vacation. Every single minute the body parts use between two to five and one-half calories. If people know that they will lose lean tissue, they may not wish to skip breakfast. Maybe they will find out that breakfast is important and allow time for it and have the food available. Maybe they will find out that eating breakfast also keeps them thin.

Skipping breakfast or any other meal day after day can result in malnutrition and eventually precipitate a medical crisis. Most people think of malnutrition as something that happens only to starving people. Malnutrition as defined in the *Dictionary of Medical Practice*[3] is: "the condition caused by the improper balance between what a individual eats and what he requires to maintain health." Malnutrition can be the result of a diet that has an incorrect balance of the basic nutrients, either too much or too little of fat, protein, carbohydrates, minerals, vitamins. It can arise from malabsorption of digested food or from a metabolic malfunction of one or more parts of the body.

When the body is low on fuel, the parts that are cannibalized first are those that are the most vulnerable because of genetics or a trauma . . . an operation or an injury. Damaged lean cells, more than healthy cells, means that there are less cells to do the work and fewer cells to pick up the glucose and store glucose as glycogen. The person may need to consume starch carbohydrates more often throughout the day. How many people complain of an old injury hurting at certain times? Is the reason it hurts because they have been skipping meals or consuming less calories than their lean tissue cell weight demands? Consider the results and imagine the possible long-term effects on health of skipping meals or consuming too few calories:

Loss of Lean Tissue

A lose of lean tissue may cause the following:

- The heart rate may slow becoming arrhythmic (skip beats).
- Body temperature may drop even with excess body fat insulation.
- Blood cholesterol may rise.
- Toxins become more potent.
- Diabetes may become a higher risk.
- Development of diverticulitis, diarrhea or constipation may occur.
- Kidney and bladder stones may develop after following a low calorie diet.
- Osteoporosis becomes a greater risk.
- The immune system may have difficulty fighting off infections and diseases such as multiple sclerosis, lupus, arthritis, allergies, fibromyalgia and cancer.
- The thyroid gland may shrink causing the body temperature to drop, hair to fall out and/or become gray and mousy looking, the nails may peel and body fat may increase.
- The risk for a stroke or heart attack is increased because the blood may thicken.
- Development of bronchitis, emphysema or lung cancer is greater.
- Medications may become toxic.
- Women can stop menstruating and men can become impotent.
- Confusion or forgetfulness may occur.
- A skin rash can develop.
- Gums can bleed and teeth may fall out.
- Irritability may become more prominent.
- If a pregnancy occurs the unborn child can be hurt.
- With inadequate calories, the dominos fall.

With less cells the different parts of the body give off warnings. But people may ignore them because they lack the understanding, or every day pressures keep them from doing something about it, or they think the sign or symptom is minor and will go away.

Case in Point

A woman was diagnosed with Ehlers-Danlos syndrome, a deterioration of the muscles and connective tissues. She reported that she jogged each day and that for the past few years her leg muscles had become progressively weaker, as did other muscles in her body. A specialist, she said, claimed nutrition would not help.

As the disease progressed, she needed more medication to relieve the pain. She had read about the benefits of positive thinking and consulted a psychologist. When she asked her about nutrition, the woman was referred to me.

This woman was the top saleswoman for a national company. She had become involved in her employees' lives, helped them over stumbling blocks to their own successes, and generated enthusiasm. But she told me she would forget to eat for 24 to 48 hours.

This lifestyle kept her very thin, but no one had pointed out to her the consequences of not eating. She assumed that the fat on her body or the food she would eat several days later would make up for her lack of calories. She did not realize that this routine most likely was being conducted at the expense of her muscles and connective tissues. She showed me how she could twist her finger around unconditionally, as well as separate her shoulder from her arm muscle. She lifted her blouse to reveal two hollows in her back where muscles once were. I assumed that her connective tissue and muscles had been sacrificed to provide the blood glucose necessary to operate the vital parts of her body such as her brain, nerves, heart and lungs.

I thought that if she ate enough calories and nutrients spread over three meals and a snack that some of the muscles and connective tissues would return. Fortunately, most of them did. Her caloric needs were based on her lean tissue and body fat weight, with calories added for insulation, exercise and illness. I used the computer to design a menu that would provide 2600 calories or 800 calories per meal.

Realistically, with her busy schedule, how was she ever going to put these meal plans into practice? Where would she find time to buy the food and prepare the meals? Could she adjust her schedule?

Her husband, who worked with her in the business, was a gourmet cook and volunteered to put the meals in front of her. We regularly reviewed what she recorded for her food intake, discussed recipes, shopping, and eating in hotels, airplanes, cars. Each week as she gained more strength, she became more motivated and adhered more to the meal plan. Within six months, she was no longer taking medication, was unable to twist her finger or separate her shoulder. The hollows in her back filled in. Her connective tissue disease is under control. But even though this story appears to have a happy ending, this woman still struggles with dietary discipline every day.

Saving Lean Tissue

If people heed the warnings that they experience from their bodies, they may be able to prevent the loss of lean tissue cells and, thus, health can be saved. You probably have heard it over and over again. "Catch it in the bud" or "The sooner you pay attention to warnings, the better chance you have of recovery." What significantly impacts on our health are our lifestyle decisions. These decisions begin with nutritional practices. The first decision may be to eat breakfast every day. Other decisions may be to eliminate common undesirable substances in the diet and the environment, to reduce body fat, to gain lean weight and, of course, to exercise. Every part of the body is important and the cells that comprise the body parts need a constant supply of nutrients and calories three to four times daily. Our body parts are always working. They are never on vacation.

Chapter Notes:

1: The *circumference measurement* uses a measuring tape. It is the simplest, the most workable, and the easiest for recording changes, whether the person is young or old, thin or obese. The formula converts measurements into constants and arrives at a percent body fat. For years, the Dairy and Nutrition Council, Inc, published this formula in its booklet for adolescents. *Underwater weighing* is called the gold standard for determining our body fat and against which all other devices are measured. One sits on a scale seat and is lowered into a tank. The principle is based on the idea that fat floats. The more body fat one has, the more one's body floats to the top. A scale records the amount. However, underwater weighing is inconvenient for tracking one's lean tissue on a weekly basis. *Bio-electric Impedance Analysis* is a device in which electrodes are placed on one's wrist and ankle. A very low electric current is sent through the body. The current picks up the body's potassium levels. A computer registers the amount and this is represents one's lean tissue weight. However, the results lack accuracy. They can vary with a person's skin temperature, room temperature, time of last meal, and body position. *Calipers* have been used for years, are simple, and inexpensive. The calipers are used to measure body fat in various locations on the body. The operator's fingers pull up some fat away from the lean tissue, squeezes the calipers over the fat and records it. Using these figures and a formula, body fat is calculated. Several problems arise. The amount of fat pulled up can vary from one moment to the next. No two people arrive at the same measurement because the operators can exert various pressures when squeezing the calipers. It is difficult to pull body fat away from the lean on obese and overweight people and on children. It is difficult not to pull up some lean tissue with the fat on elderly people. *Body Mass Index* (BMI) measures body fat in pounds but is not refined enough to measure for changes in body fat and lean tissue cells on a weekly basis.

2: The standard system for determining calories uses .8 grams of protein per kilogram of total weight. The system, I used is 1.4 grams of protein per kilogram of *lean tissue weight*.

3: The following example will show how to calculate your calories.

Robin (total wt = 135lbs)
Her lean weight is 115lbs
Divide 115lbs by 2.2 = 52 Kg
52 Kg x 1.4 = 72 gms protein
72 gms x 4 = 291 calories
291 x 6.5 = 1892 calories
* Robin will need 1892 calories
(Using protein as 15% of the total)

Gary (total wt = 170lbs)
His lean weight is 140lbs
Divide 140lbs by 2.2 = 63 Kg
63 Kg x 1.4 = 88 gms protein
88 gms x 4 = 352 calories
352 x 6.5 = 2288 calories
* Gary will need 2288 calories

CHAPTER 2

The Cell Is Like A Factory
When Raw Materials Are Short,
The Managers Steal And Fight

JEFF wanted to lose weight and had put himself on a liquid diet of 400 to 500 calories a day. A few weeks later, he experienced blurred vision. His doctor reported that Jeff's blood glucose was extremely high, diagnosed diabetes, prescribed insulin, and referred him to me.

I measured him for body fat and lean tissue and determined that he needed at least 1800 calories a day. He followed the meal plan and his eyesight improved. His blood glucose dropped to a normal level almost immediately. Within three weeks, his eyesight was normal. Four months later, he was off insulin. And he lost weight—on 1800 calories a day.

Lean tissue is made up of cells—75 to 100 trillion in an adult, depending on the person and on which research source is cited. Each of our cells can grow, metabolize, reproduce, and respond to stimuli if it has enough glucose and nutrients. Additionally, many kinds of substances and events can interfere with a cell's ability to receive or accept enough glucose and nutrients, compromising the cell's performance. The cell can be cannibalized to provide energy.

Let me explain. The body is comprised of 200 types of cells. Each set of cells performs specific jobs. For instance, the brain, weighing in at three pounds, is comprised of 100 billion nerve cells (neurons), and a trillion support cells.

As the cells use up their energy (glucose) and nutrients, they need to be renourished to continue working efficiently. In any one instant, several trillion cells are at the "trough" (the blood stream) being refueled. But not all the cells rejuvenate at one time. While some are refueling, others are working. The time it takes for all the cells in the set to refuel is called the *turnover rate.*

As an example, the trillion cells in the immune system group take 12 hours to turn over completely. This group refuels more often than any other. When there is a deficit of glucose or nutrients in the blood, the immune system is one of the first to be affected. The 60 billion cells in the eyes take 24 hours to turn over. The trillion cells in each of the intestinal tracts take 48 hours to completely turn over. Red blood cells take several weeks, and bones several months. As the body ages, these turnover rates slow because there are fewer cells—and thus less lean tissue—to perform. How carefully and regularly the body is fed, impacts significantly on health later in life.

Cells receive their glucose and nutrients from the blood stream. The blood stream receives them from the intestinal tract which is the processing plant. That is, the intestinal tract digests and breaks down your food to single molecules. The single molecules are absorbed into the blood stream which carries them to all the cells, like a tree whose roots absorb nutrients and water from the soil and distribute them to each leaf. If the intestinal tract's function is impaired, cells throughout the body can starve.

Each cell has a nucleus which controls how much and what it accepts. Therefore, the amount of nutrients taken up from the blood stream by the cell is programmed and limited. The more cells you have, the more calories and nutrients you need.

Your cells can be compared to a factory where fuel and raw materials are needed to produce a product. In a factory, the fuel may be gas or oil and the raw materials may be cotton, wool, wood, steel, plastic, chemicals, etc. Fuel provides the energy for the machinery to use the raw materials and create the product. In the factory, as the fuel combusts with oxygen and creates the energy, waste products, carbon monoxide, carbon, and other chemicals are expelled through the chimney.

A similar action takes place in your body.

The fuel is macro-nutrients—protein, carbohydrates and fat which contain calories. The main fuel is carbohydrates which convert 100 percent in the intestinal tract to glucose. The micro-nutrients are vitamins, minerals, water, and oxygen, none of which *provide calories or energy*. Even so, they are needed in the presence of hormones and enzymes to convert the macro-nutrients into energy. The micro-nutrients are, in this illustration, the raw materials. Between them, products are created. The body functions: the eyes see, the heart beats, the brain thinks, the muscles move, etc. These actions produce waste products-water and carbon dioxide. Water is excreted through the kidneys and bladder and evaporates from skin, lungs, eyes, mouth, and nose. Carbon dioxide is excreted through the lungs.

What Is a Macro Without a Micro

To work efficiently, your cells need all 60 of the nutrients that the macro—and micro-nutrients provide. Some nutrients which the body must never be without are stored by specific cells. For instance, your fat cells store fat; muscle cells store glucose as glycogen. Your liver cells are "programmed" to store copper, glucose, and vitamins A and D. Bone cells are "programmed" to pick up and store more calcium than other cells. Since amino acids and water soluble vitamins are not stored, they must come from food every few hours.

Sugar, An Oxymoron

Food is defined as something which contains calories and nutrients to nourish and sustain the body's energy. Applying this definition, can sugar and alcohol be considered food when neither contain any nutrients? Yet, when they enter the body they must be processed by nutrients. The nutrients are taken from other cells which use them to keep us healthy. Therefore, sugar and alcohol can be considered bandits because they steal from our cells and interfere with the cells' performance.

Remember the report from Cuba which cited the neurological and vision problems in sugar cane workers whose main diet was the sugar they harvested in the fields? A similar situation occurred in India when brown rice was refined to white rice robbing it of thiamin and other nutrients. Closer to home, soft drinks are a typical American favorite source. In one extreme case a woman lived on soda pop and became unable to eat food. She bled from various parts of her body and became very anemic.

Why do some people become sick from sugar? If sugar is the primary source of energy, the body becomes nutritionally depleted. Sugar is a simple carbohydrate without other nutrients, whereas, foods from the starch group are complex carbohydrates which contain nutrients.

All carbohydrates are digested to glucose in the intestinal tract. In converting the glucose to energy, the cells need oxygen and vitamins. One of the vitamins it needs is thiamin, a B vitamin. The amount of thiamin needed is in direct proportion to the amount of carbohydrate ingested. Since thiamin is a water-soluble vitamin that cannot be stored, it must accompany the carbohydrates into the stomach which it does with complex carbohydrates. But sugar comes calling empty-handed. Some people may jump to the conclusion that all they need to do is to take thiamin in supplement form. But thiamin alone cannot solve the problem. It too interacts with other nutrients, enzymes and hormones.

The No Nutrient Twins: Sugar and Alcohol

Two other nutrients which sugar and alcohol rob from the body are copper and chromium. The body does store some in the liver, but the amount is limited and can be used up. The need for chromium more than doubles and the need for copper triples with the ingestion of alcohol or sugar! Therefore the more sugar or alcohol you consume the faster the copper and chromium supplies are depleted. If chromium is depleted diabetes may develop. When copper is depleted, blood cholesterol can rise. This obviously is not good news for those consuming products stripped of fat and enhanced by sugar.

Exactly which cells give up which nutrients vary with each person from time to time, and from meal to meal. Sugar and alcohol can contribute to one person's adding fat to their body, to another's anemia, another's headache, another's irritability, and another's illness or disease, or can interfere with a child's growth. An example of what can happen did happen—to Molly.

Eight-year-old Molly, who was referred to me by my husband, had been placed in a classroom for children with Attention Deficit Disorder. A pediatrician, he believed that diet was interfering with Molly's concentration. A computer analysis of her food intake revealed her sugar consumption was high. Her eating habits included sugar-coated cereals and toast with jelly for breakfast, fruit packed in syrup, cookies, gelatin in the school lunch menu, and ice cream and Kool-Aid for dinner. She said she had a hard time staying awake in class. I provided her with a systematic plan of nutritious foods to support her growing body and her mother said she would help Molly follow it. The child was to eliminate sugar for one week to see if there would be a change in her behavior. Several days later, the teacher reported to the mother that Molly was more attentive and alert in class. But that weekend, Molly attended a birthday party where her mother later found her asleep in a corner. She had eaten ice cream and cake.

In another instance I provided a meal plan for a woman who was depressed and didn't like the side effects of tranquilizers. Her meals had consisted of two to three candy bars daily, cookies and cake and in between six bottles of caffeinated soda pop "to give me energy." When she followed a systematic meal plan of nutritious foods to support her lean tissue cells and eliminated the sugar and caffeine, she said she was amazed at her increased energy, heightened mental attitude, and elimination of nightmares. She later reported she had weaned herself from the tranquilizers and has had only a few episodes of depression.

Several others have told me that when they consume sugar, sugar substitutes or alcohol, they are more tired or hyperactive, less alert, more depressed, and sometimes ache or develop an infection. I believe that in such cases the cells' ability to perform has been compromised.

For those who add body fat easily, sugar and sugar substitutes can add it faster than dietary fat. Sugar and sugar substitutes turn on the insulin hormone. Dietary fat does not.

Low-Fat, No-Fat Diets

What a shocking statement! Of course, it is true that many people eat too much fat and too many calories, both of which can create serious health problems. People have been bombarded with this message for years and are ready to surrender to the low-fat and fat-free messages. Food manufacturers have moved in on this territory and are fanning the fat free frenzy and profiting. In 1991-1992 alone, they introduced 2500 new fat-free or low-fat products. People are buying them because they may not be sure how much fat they should consume and may reason "why not just choose foods with little or no fat and then we can be healthier and thinner."

Fat Free Products

However, how do these products taste without fat? When the fat disappears from the product, so does the flavor. To compensate, sugar and/or salt often are added. For instance, low-fat turkey and roast beef from the delicatessen each have several hundred milligrams more of sodium per serving than raw turkey or raw lean ground round beef. Low-fat salad dressings have much more sodium than oil and vinegar dressing. A person who is sensitive to sodium can accumulate as much as eight pounds of water overnight.

A patient told me that she went to a party where salted popcorn was served before dinner. She was so hungry she ate several cups full. Being obsessed with her weight she weighed herself morning and night. Before going to bed that night she weighed four pounds more than she had in the morning. The next morning she weighed an additional four pounds. She was puffy. Many people tell me they are aware when have consumed too much sodium. Their shoes will be too tight or they can not remove the rings from their fingers. A high intake of sodium can mean trouble for those with kidney problems and high blood pressure. Extra dietary sodium also can also trigger the excretion of calcium and thereby increase the risk for osteoporosis.

Sugar has its own problems. When it is added to foods, calories are added. For instance, low fat yogurt often has as many calories as high-fat ice cream. Low fat cookies often have as many calories as the high-fat variety. What takes only one high fat cookie to make you feel satisfied takes a whole box of the low-fat variety and you have eaten 20 times more calories. But since people are buying into the idea that it is fat, not sugar, that makes them fat and raises their blood cholesterol, they ignore the sugar content.

Fat fearers often complain of fatigue and hunger. Neither their energy or their satisfaction is sustained by the sugary foods. They keep wanting more. They may develop characteristics similar to those of an anorexic. They become obsessed with food, opening and closing the refrigerator door, searching the kitchen cupboards for something to eat, or grazing continuously after three o'clock in the afternoon. Up until this time they have been able to resist foods with fat, but when night arrives, they are hungry and ready for a big meal and give in and eat some fat. At last, they are satisfied.

So which should people be more concerned about in products: the fat content or the sugar/salt content? For many Americans, the low-fat, no-fat diet is the diet of choice. But what does it do for their health? People unknowingly may be squeezing their meals and foods dry and putting their lean tissue and thus their health at risk. Consider the following.

Are people losing weight? Which kind—body fat or lean tissue? Are they replacing the fat calories with complex carbohydrates? If not, their calories may be too low. How does a low-fat, no-fat diet affect the mucous membranes, the immune system, the liver and the bones? Do health professionals who recommend that people consume only 10 to 15 percent of the calories in fat in their diets also sound a note of warning? Is there any mention of *inadequate* fat consumption in this country?

It may be hard to believe, but dietary fat is as important as any of the other nutrients—the vitamins, minerals, protein and carbohydrates. Fat adds a delicious taste, satisfaction and aroma to foods and meals and keeps the food moist. In the body, fat carries the fat soluble vitamins from the intestinal tract to the liver. It slows the progress of food through the intestinal tract so that the enzymes can digest the food.

Susie had high blood cholesterol. She was told by the staff in her physician's office to reduce the amount of fat and cholesterol she was consuming. After several months, when her blood cholesterol did not drop, her doctor wanted to prescribe a medication—but she refused. Instead, she continued to reduce her fat intake to 6 grams a day which, of course, also meant that her caloric intake was reduced to 800 calories. Finally, after a year without any improvement in her blood cholesterol she consented to take the medication. The particular medication prescribed for her prevented the absorption of fat. Three weeks later, her eye hemorrhaged. I agreed it could have been from the medication but I also believed that her nearly fat-free diet was suspect.

Fat Soluble Vitamins

The fat soluble vitamins are A, D, E and K. When dietary fat is inadequate, fat soluble vitamins are not absorbed and lean tissue cells are lost. A person who has not been absorbing fat soluble vitamins may gain weight, feel very tired, have dry or brittle hair, cracked and bleeding fingers, lingering colds or coughs or high blood cholesterol.

People may not connect their consumption of too little fat with the symptoms and signs mentioned above because it takes weeks or months of a low-fat, no-fat diet to deplete the body of fat soluble vitamins. Unlike water soluble vitamins, fat-soluble vitamins are stored and released slowly. But at some point, if a low-fat, no-fat diet continues, one or more symptoms or signs will appear. Then health is impaired. Lean-tissue cells have been lost. For instance, you can lose bone cells and not even know it.

But once you consume enough calories, fat and nutrients to support your lean tissue, many cells return. The body is a marvelous piece of machinery and can recover fairly well. Research bears this out. However, it means bucking the low-fat, no-fat tide.

Lubricating Lean Tissue Cells with Vitamin A

Certain cells cannot perform when the fat soluble vitamins are not available. Consider vitamin A. This is not to say that vitamins D, K, and E are any less important, but they are discussed in chapters 4, 8, and 9.

Vitamin A is so important to the performance of the lean tissue cells that the liver cells store it for the time when it is not included in the diet. The functions of vitamin A and another form of vitamin A, carotene, are to keep the immune system healthy, to build bone and to keep the mucous membrane cells moist and healthy.

Mucous membranes are everywhere (See Chapter Notes). They are the barrier between irritants such as bacteria, acids, and other chemicals and the inner parts, the blood stream and the nerves. Picture the mucus as analogous to the bubble or foam we wrap around precious china and glassware to protect them. The bubble wrap contains trapped air as the cushion.

Mucous membranes contain water that protects the precious blood vessels and nerves. If the mucous membranes become dry, the nerves can be exposed and cause pain. If the blood vessels are exposed, they bleed.

If the mucous lining in the intestinal tract begins to dry up from the lack of vitamin A, the number of enzymes to digest foods is reduced or is lost. Those enzymes may be the ones that digest wheat, lactose, raw vegetables or fruits. The undigested food is left in the intestinal tract causing still further problems. It ferments, "scratches" and irritates causing gas, bloating, diarrhea, constipation, bleeding and/or pain. Since the intestinal tract is the gateway to the rest of the cells in the body, the whole body suffers when it does not receive enough vitamin A.

Vitamin A can be stored in the liver but since there is no gauge, there will be no warning when the liver finally runs out of it. Then suddenly one day these problems arise:

- Break through bleeding which can occur anywhere in the body, and the person becomes anemic and tired.

- The eye can die if mucous membranes surrounding it dry up and hemorrhage.

- Infections can enter dry mucous membranes—ears, sinus cavities, lungs, and bronchial tubes. Air that is too dry or a diet too low in fat or by both can dry out mucous membranes

- The lining surrounding the bladder can dry up, causing excruciating pain, then bacteria can enter.

- The immune system may break down, resulting in auto immune diseases or making it possible for cancer to invade the cells.

- Bones can deteriorate.

Many times people react to these symptoms by either seeking the help of a doctor who may prescribe a medication, or they may decide to take supplements, but rarely do they think their "healthy" low-fat, no-fat diet is the basic problem.

Vitamin A Sources

When people believe that a vitamin A supplement will solve their problem, they may not know of its dangers. In one report alone, a Philadelphia hospital recorded 21 cases of vitamin A toxicity over a period of three years. The toxicity occurred with supplements, not with food. The Recommended Daily Allowance (RDA) (See Appendix D) is for only 5000 I.U. a day.[4] Yet there are people ingesting from 10,000 to 50,000 I.U. for skin problems, acne, hair loss, dry skin, eyesight, or allergies. The symptoms of toxicity are similar to those that vitamin A is supposed to prevent (See Chapter 10).

A mother called me because her beautiful daughter of 14 was losing her hair. Her daughter flipped her long hair forward so that I could see the bare spots on her head. Her mother was giving her 50,000 I.U. of vitamin A. But when I analyzed her food intake she was only consuming about 10 grams of fat. She drank skim milk, ate white chicken and fish, fruits and vegetables, dry bread, rice and noodles, but no butter, margarine or oil. When I tried to explain to the mother that 50,000 units of vitamin A was too much and was probably causing her daughter's hair loss, she said that it wasn't the vitamin A. When I suggested that she increase the amount of fat in her daughter's diet so that fat soluble vitamins could be absorbed, she became irate. She did not want her daughter to like the high-fat foods because she might develop high-blood cholesterol. If any of the above problems are experienced taking a medication may mask the underlying cause or even add to upheaval. A dietary analysis may reveal whether your fat intake is too low. You can recover by adding to your diet a little more fat, foods with vitamin A and a few more servings of starches. This will fuel the performance of lean tissue cells.

Good Foods are Available

With our current supply, is it possible for people to find the foods they need to protect their lean tissue cells?

You bet it is. The markets have wonderful life-giving foods which contain all the macro-and micro-nutrients in their natural state. Can people develop the necessary discipline to follow a regime? Many of my students and patients have. Maybe people just need to be given permission to eat if they have not been eating enough to feed their lean tissue cells, or they need the discipline to eat meals on time and choose life giving foods.

Jason was six years old when I first saw him in 1995. His mother reported that he had had earaches, sinus problems, colds, infections and allergies since he was two years of age. Regularly for those four years he was given an antibiotic, an inhaler, and allergy medication. He was absent a great deal from school. The school teacher suggested that the mother seek my advice.

Jason appeared to be dehydrated, withdrawn, pale and malnourished with dark circles under his eyes. His mother reported that he snored at night, that his ears were blocked and he could not pass a hearing test, had headaches and sometimes vomited. He weighed 46 pounds.

I provided Jason with a computerized meal plan based on his lean weight and growth needs. The meal plan incorporated the "Safe Diet" foods because I believed his intestinal tract was affected by all the medications. Our goal? Within two weeks, Jason was to be consuming 2200 calories of which 40 to 45 percent would be made up of fat. The first three meals were hard for him to eat, but with encouragement from his mother he began to eat more. Within ten days Jason was so hungry between meals that he was consuming more than 2400 calories. In three weeks, he was able to eliminate two medications, was not coughing, was sleeping through the night without snoring, and he was smiling and appeared happy.

By process of elimination, his mother and I figured out that Jason could drink skim milk. He always complained of a headache after he drank homogenized milk, but not when he drank skim milk. Because of his allergies, his parents installed a new furnace for cleaner air. By the fourth week, he had eliminated all but one medication. His hearing test was normal, much to the astonishment of his physician. In the eighth and 16th weeks, everyone around him had a cold but his body was able to fight it off. And without medication. After being on the "Safe Diet" for 16 weeks he gained three pounds. His mother reported he did not seem to have any asthma. In 1996, I talked to his mother. She reported that their medical bills had dropped 95 percent and that Jason was growing, playing soccer and was very healthy.

Because Jason complained of his stomach and sometimes vomited, I provided him with a "Safe Diet" (See Appendix). His intestinal tract needed to recover before it could properly work. Otherwise, how could he receive enough macro- and micro-nutrients so necessary to repair his lungs, ears, nose, and immune system?

The intestinal tract is the gateway to the rest of the body and central to the processing of food. How carefully the intestinal tract cells are fed can impact on health significantly.

Chapter Notes:

1: Sources of Chromium: liver, brewer's yeast, whole grains, wheat germ, nuts, broccoli, asparagus, cheese, prunes, mushrooms, and wine and beer that have been prepared in steel vats. Chromium has been processed out of white flour and white rice so products without yeast like crackers, pretzels, pasta, biscuits, muffins have no chromium. Whole wheat bread with yeast has chromium as does brown rice. A cheese (real cheese, not imitation) sandwich or pizza made with whole wheat flour has chromium. If you want to be a little original, sprinkle a tablespoon or two of wheat germ on the whole grain cereal each morning. This will provide enough chromium for the day.

2: Sources of copper are: shellfish, liver, kidney, nuts, legumes, raisins, cocoa and green leafy vegetables grown in copper-rich soil.

3: Mucous membranes are everywhere in our bodies. Their primary purpose is to provide moisture and a cushion to protect the eyes, ears, nose, mouth, lungs, esophagus, and trachea, intestinal track, bladder, kidneys, vagina, urethra, and prostate. Without fat and therefore, without vitamin A, the mucous membranes dry up.

- Eyes can become blurred and hemorrhage
- Ears can become infected, even though an antibiotic is given repeatedly.
- Persistent infections in the sinuses and bronchial tubes can cause coughing, pain and runny rose.
- Allergies can appear.
- The mouth can develop sores.
- The esophagus and trachea can begin to bleed.
- The lungs can be susceptible to pneumonia.
- The bladder can be susceptible to cystitis.
- The hair can become brittle and lackluster.
- The skin can develop rashes or sores or become dry.
- The intestinal tract can develop yeast infections, spasms of diarrhea or constipation because it lacks lubrication and may not produce some enzymes. Fiber, lactose, and gluten can become irritants. Couple the dry mucous cells that line the intestinal tract with antibiotics or any medication that irritates, and the 'bad' bacteria in the colon may overwhelm the 'good' bacteria and death can result.

4: Vitamin A, is found in animal foods: butter, cheese, milk, eggs yolks, cod liver oil, and liver. A *Synthetic* vitamin A is added to such foods as skim milk and margarine, but, if packaged in opaque material and exposed to light, whether in the dairy cases or in the refrigerator, up to 40 percent of the vitamin A can be lost. Milk, cheese, and yogurt should be purchased in paper cartons.

Carotene is found in orange and dark green vegetables and fruits such as cantaloupe, sweet potatoes, carrots, spinach, broccoli, greens, etc. Carotene is converted in the liver to vitamin A. But for the vitamin A or carotene to be absorbed fat must travel with these foods through the intestinal tract.

CHAPTER 3

The Intestinal Tract
The Processing Plant For Fuel

THE intestinal tract is the gateway to the rest of the body. If it is in trouble, the body is in trouble. If the intestinal tract is not well nourished, or is receiving too much food but not the right kind, it cannot process or produce as much energy as it should. Since more than half of the population in the United States has intestinal problems, then half the population is unhealthy.

Proof of the numbers is reflected on the shelves of over-the-counter medications; the largest niche in the grocery store next to food and beverages. Add the drugs prescribed for serious gastrointestinal problems such as heartburn, ulcers, hiatus hernia, reflux, Irritable Bowel Syndrome, food intolerances and acid stomach and it becomes obvious that Americans are spending at a runaway rate just to fix that part of their bodies that processes food. The 1992 sales, for instance, reported by the makers of just two prescription drugs, Zantac and Tagamet were $4.5 billion.

Instead of drugs which may mask or aggravate the problem, why not find the causes first? It may be the result of one or more of the following: not enough food, too much food, an allergy, a food intolerance, or interference from medications or other substances. Making and keeping an appointment with a gastroenterologist would be one of the first steps for a person whose intestinal tract is in trouble. A specialist such as this can rule out a bacterial or virus infection, a parasitic infestation, cancer or some other serious problem. You should not wait when you have intestinal problems. Delay can mean further damage, some of it unrepairable.

If no problem is found, identifying and eliminating the offending substance in food and beverages is next. Keeping a diary is the best method. One can record, over a period of two weeks every food, beverage or ingredient that enters the mouth, at what time and then note the body's reaction (See Appendix D for an example).

The suspected offending substance then can be eliminated for two weeks, consumed again and the reaction recorded. This process can be repeated until one is convinced that the culprit has been identified. Primary suspects are alcohol, vitamins, caffeine, sugar, medications. Other possibilities are food intolerances such as lactose, plant oils, fruits, vegetables, allergies, and additives (See Chapter Notes).

One of my patients complained of flatulence (gas). I suggested she record what she ate and drank for two weeks. She noted that every afternoon a half hour after she ate a banana, the flatulence came back. So she eliminated the bananas for several weeks and substituted nectarines, grapes or peaches instead. As time went on she became more convinced that bananas were the offending substance, because each time she ate a banana, the flatulence returned. Believing she could never have a banana again, she went without them for two years. Then one day she was tempted to try a piece. No flatulence. She gradually added it to her diet and now, three years later, she is able to eat a half of a banana with no problems.

Flatulence or gas results from the fermentation and accumulation of water in the intestinal tract because the intestinal tract is not digesting the food. It is enzymes produced in the mucous membrane of the marvelously engineered intestinal tract which digest the food. The lining of the intestinal tract produces thousands of enzymes. The enzymes digest food to single molecules of nutrients (See Chapter Notes). The single molecules then pass into the blood stream which carries the nutrients to the 75 trillion cells. The mucous cells also act as a barrier from damaging chemicals and bacteria which you may ingest. The cells in the mucous membrane are constantly sloughing off and are renewed as they receive enough calories and nutrients. The amount of energy that the intestinal tract uses in a day is not much—only ten percent or about 200 calories (based on a 2000 calorie diet). But the intestinal tract does not have priority for the available calories.

If the body does not receive enough calories and nutrients, the cells in the intestinal tract and the mucous membranes can be the lean tissue which is recruited and converted to glucose. With less cells, the mucous membranes can become thin and easily violated. A thinner mucous membrane produces less enzymes. When food is not digested, it damages cells as the muscles push the food through the intestinal tract. Irritated cells lead to diarrhea, constipation, flatulence, cramping and bloating. With more damaged cells, fewer single molecule nutrients are available to reach the blood stream. The body receives less glucose from food and more from lean tissue cells. With thinner mucous membrane barriers, the underlying cells can be damaged by chemicals, bacteria, undigested food and toxins.

Therefore another step in analyzing the cause of intestinal problems is to ask, "Are enough calories and nutrients, divided into meals, being consumed every five hours?"

Allergies Versus Food Intolerances

Allergies can trigger intestinal problems. They can easily be confused with food intolerances because diarrhea can occur in both. Diarrhea needs to be treated and the cause identified. When food travels through the intestinal tract without being digested the body becomes malnourished. Because treatment for allergies and food intolerances differ, it is important to distinguish between them. An allergist can test for antibody production. Then the substance can be eliminated and a medication given to reduce the allergic reaction.

Many adults believe they are allergic to a food, but tests do not reveal it. Maybe they were told as a child that they were allergic to milk. But now they can drink it. Perhaps the intestinal tract and immune system just needed time to mature. Usually tests for food allergies are not reliable because people react to various foods on a day to day basis. Only one percent of adults and three percent of children have clinically proven allergies from food. Peanuts, eggs, soy, fish, wheat and milk have been identified as producing the most allergic reactions.

Positively identifying a food intolerance, a more common occurrence, is a bit more difficult. With the intestinal tract producing thousands of enzymes, something is bound to go wrong along the 30 foot route at some time. A food intolerance may occur only occasionally as when a person consumes too much of a certain food, too often or too many days in a row. For instance, you may have heard of someone who ate three to four green apples and then complained of a stomach ache. In this case, the enzyme production may have been overwhelmed and did not match the amount of apples being ingested. If this type of experience occurs only once in while, the intestinal tract will recover in a few days. But if the problem continues, the offending substance must be identified, eliminated or a matching enzyme added to the diet or you can become malnourished (See Chapter Notes for offending substances). More foods end up undigested causing irritation and gastrointestinal problems.

The Enzyme to Digest Lactose

The major complaint by people is the inability to digest milk. In fact, about 75 percent of the world adult population, including 40 to 50 million Americans, cannot drink milk, because their intestinal tract is missing or producing little of the lactase enzyme.

Lactase is produced in the lining of the small intestine. It digests lactose, a carbohydrate in milk, into two single molecules. It is a delicate enzyme for the intestinal tract to produce, particularly in infants and the elderly. When lactose is not digested, it remains in the intestinal tract, fermenting and attracting water about 30 minutes after being ingested. The abdomen rises like bread. Weight increases. Clothing and belts feel tighter, as was the case with Quincy.

Quincy wanted to lose weight. She was provided with a meal plan that included foods from the milk group. This was a food she did not ordinarily consume. Within a week, she complained of bloating, tight skirts, an uncomfortable stomach, and an increase in weight. I surmised that her intestinal tract lacked the enzyme to digest lactose. When she added a lactase enzyme to her meals, the bloating disappeared. She lost four pounds of water overnight and experienced an increase in energy.

Sometimes the problem of digesting milk does not appear until a person has been following a low-fat diet. Fat slows the transit time through the intestinal tract and allows more time for the enzymes, like the lactase enzyme, to digest food. In this case, chocolate, two percent, or whole milk would be better than skim milk.

The digestion of lactose is much more difficult after surgery or an accident, during an illness and while taking an antibiotic. In these cases foods with lactose should be eliminated until the intestinal tract processes return to normal.

Mark came to me for a diet to clear up his diarrhea and bloating which he believed began after he took a course of antibiotics for a cold. He also complained about a backache. When he eliminated the lactose from his diet, the diarrhea stopped, his stomach was not bloated and his back stopped aching.

Usually, the first thing people think of doing when they cannot tolerate lactose is to eliminate all foods from the milk group. But without the milk group, calcium and riboflavin are lacking and you cannot substitute another food group. The need to eliminate milk products is no longer necessary because there are products on the market which are reduced in lactose and still contain the original nutrients. The products are reduced lactose milks and yogurts, real cheese and dry cottage cheese, which contain no lactose naturally and a commercial lactase enzyme tablet which can be ingested with lactose-containing foods.

Other food products may simulate milk and cheese and have no lactose. Products such as imitation cheeses and milks pass as real food because they look, smell, and taste like the real thing. They are not the same. More importantly, they lack the milk nutrients. Imitation cheeses are served in many restaurants and on pizzas because they cost less. Sometimes they are added to frozen or packaged dishes. They are listed on the package under ingredients. Hard and natural cheeses are recommended because they contain all the *Milk Group* nutrients except lactose. The liquid whey contains lactose but it has been drained away (See Chapter Notes). The whey or lactose is commercially dried and sold to pharmaceutical manufacturers and food companies as an instant dissolving agent. (It is listed under ingredients on the label of a container as "whey protein" or lactose). Pharmaceutical manufacturers have added it to more than a thousand medications because the lactose carries the medication from the intestinal tract into the blood stream. The most common medications with lactose are antibiotics, estrogen and anti-inflammatory drugs "Contains lactose" will be listed under ingredients on the insert which accompanies all medications. Sometimes, the first indication of lactose intolerance is ingesting a medication with lactose. A pharmacist may be able to suggest a substitute medication without lactose.

The Enzyme to Digest Gluten

Another enzyme that some people lose is the enzyme to digest gluten, a protein in wheat, barley, rye and oats. This enzyme must be present for bread to rise (See Chapter Notes). The undigested gluten irritates and flattens the mucous membranes in the intestinal tract. The flattened cells cannot produce enzymes to digest fat, lactose, sucrose (sugar), minerals and water soluble vitamins. Fat is the most difficult to digest. When fat is not absorbed neither are the fat soluble vitamins, precipitating further breakdown of the mucous membranes. The result is diarrhea with the feces full of fat which float on the surface of the toilet. Without the nutrients and glucose, lean tissue cells are lost and the person loses lean tissue and becomes malnourished. The loss of lean tissue can be documented with blood tests, weight loss, hair loss, muscle, and body composition (See Chapter Notes).

For years Mary had experienced diarrhea, nausea, and cramping for years. She was depressed because she had no energy and could not stop losing weight. She said she was so discouraged about eating she was ready to commit suicide. She cried a lot. "Everything seemed to cause the diarrhea." She said she couldn't go anywhere and the various medications and enzymes prescribed by doctors had not helped. When I first met with her, she appeared to be very malnourished, very thin with a pot belly, thin legs, and wasted buttocks. Her history revealed that she also had had gall bladder and intestinal.

Her body was obviously starving to death because her intestinal tract could not digest very many foods. Most of Mary's symptoms reminded me of gluten sensitivity. Our goal was to first stop the diarrhea. I suggested that she eliminate wheat, barley, rye and oats and follow the Safe Meal Plan for one month to rebuild her body cells. That meant she had to eat and prepare all of her own foods. She agreed. I also suggested she see a gastroenterologist.

Research suggests that people who develop a sensitivity to gluten are allergic to gliadin, a constituent of gluten. The immune system responds to the presence of gliadin by destroying the enzyme that digests gluten. The number of people that develop this condition are one in 3000 people worldwide and one in 5000 people in the United States. It most likely is a genetic trait. Those of Irish descent have a risk of one in 300 and Americans with Irish ancestry may be more prone to celiac disease than Americans of other ethnic backgrounds.

In adults, this condition is usually referred to as sprue or non-tropical sprue; in children it is known as celiac disease. A gastroenterologist needs to be consulted because few people want to follow such a restrictive diet, especially if they live in the United States where the staple food is wheat. Unfortunately, there is no manmade enzyme as there is for lactose nor is there any drug that allows a person to tolerate the consumption of wheat. Once diagnosed, the person with gluten sensitivity can never again consume wheat because the danger, from a constant irritation of the intestinal tract from gluten or any other irritant, is cancer or some other very serious disease.

To prevent further damage I suggest people with gluten sensitivity follow the "Safe Diet" without the wheat, barley, rye and oats for a month or more. Then gradually introduce one food at a time (without gluten) and record the reaction. On this regime (See Appendix) people with gluten sensitivity can regain lean tissue, energy, their health and can lose excess water in their ankles. It may take from several months to a year.

As for Mary (20), the diarrhea stopped almost immediately. But whenever she ate vegetable oil, lactose, or anything with gluten, it returned.

A person with celiac disease or sprue can be diagnosed and can follow the diet. But there are people in the "gray zone" who are more difficult to diagnose because they can tolerate small amounts of wheat, once a week or once a day. However, when they eat more, they have similar symptoms usually attributed to sprue, such as sudden bouts of abdominal pain, frequent belching, gas and/ or diarrhea. Like people with sprue, they also can become malnourished. It is my belief that the mucous lining in their intestinal tract is able to produce small amounts of the enzyme to digest wheat but can't match the larger intakes. Since people in the "gray zone" do not fit the diagnosis for gluten sensitivity, they usually are diagnosed with Irritable Bowel Syndrome (IBS). Interestingly some people with IBS report being allergic to wheat as infants or as children. They can benefit from following the "Safe Diet" and gluten-free diet.

Shawn did not have the usual signs and symptoms of being wheat-sensitive. But he was extremely thin and anemic. The doctors examined his intestinal tract for the loss of blood, but could find nothing amiss. When the doctor gave me Shawn's nutritional and medical history, I found that Shawn had been ingesting large amounts of vitamin supplements, including Vitamin C, which I thought may have injured the mucous membranes in his intestinal tract. I suggested that he eliminate the vitamins supplements, vegetable fat, and lactose and follow a nutritional meal plan to support his lean tissue weight. However, after following this regime for several weeks, he remained anemic and said he felt miserable. Then I suggested that he eliminate the wheat for two weeks. He felt better instantly and decided to continue the diet without wheat. A few months later, his blood test showed a normal hemoglobin level. Six months later when he came to see me, he had gained 12 pounds, all of it lean tissue and he no longer had wasted buttocks. Incidentally, this man is of Irish descent.

The Enzyme to Digest Fat

What is not widely known is that animal and vegetable fats use different enzymes for digestion. This piece of information has helped many of my patients who have had intestinal or immune system problems. Authors Willem Linsheer and Antoine J. Vergroesen report that most texts treat the digestion of fats as one and the same, as do most brochures, medical journals, articles and other publications that focus on the intestinal tract.[5]

Butter and some animal fats are digested in the mouth and stomach to single fatty acid molecules and enter the blood stream. Whereas, vegetable fats are not digested until they reach the small intestine. Then two things must occur. First, bile must be released from the gallbladder to break down the fat into small globules. The globules must be small for the lipase enzyme, produced by the pancreas to digest the fat, to single fatty acid molecules before they can enter the lymph system, the fatty acids travel through the lymph system to the liver where they are coated with protein before they can enter the watery blood stream.

Obviously, more things can go wrong with the digestion of vegetable fats than with butter and animal fats. Age is a factor. Scientific research confirms that older adults and children, digest butter fat easier than vegetable fats.

A 13-month old baby wouldn't eat and was said to stare at the ceiling while in her crib. The mother told me that the child loved the French fries at a fast food restaurant, but not the French fries baked in the oven at home. At the time, the restaurant fried its potatoes in animal fat while the frozen variety was coated in vegetable fat. *Vegetable fats were a suspected culprit considering that the baby's intestinal tract was still developing; the enzyme may not yet have been active.* When the mother switched to preparing the child's foods with animal fat and butter and eliminated the vegetable fat, she reported that the child's normal eating and sleeping habits returned. Eventually the child's intestinal tract matured and she was able to eat vegetable fat.

Since vegetable fats have more of an opportunity to injure the intestinal tract further along, such offending substances as alcohol, antibiotics and medications can just add to an already irritated intestinal tract. Less glucose and nutrients are able to enter the blood stream and feed the cells.

Not only are the mucous membranes in the intestinal tract irritated by undigested fat and offending substances, but waste products from the breakdown of lean tissue cells irritate the kidney and bladder. The bladder is especially affected because it is a holding tank for liquid waste products. People with recurring problems of the kidney, bladder, prostate, or urinary tract may fare better if the fats they consume are butter or animal fats.

The following case was a challenge.

Clara developed polio at the age of eight and had her first (undiagnosed) attack of pancreatitis at the age of 16. At 19, she was hospitalized. She said her doctor told her she had a nervous stomach and was malnourished. At 21, pregnant with her first child, she developed gestational diabetes. After her second pregnancy she nearly died from a major pancreatic attack. In her early to mid 20's she had pneumonia twice. She had several recurring bouts of pancreatitis before she was 45. She took Pancrease to replace the enzymes her pancreas could not produce. In 1985, she said doctors estimated that her pancreas was 95 percent calcified with a prognosis of diabetes within two years. Recently, a glycosylated hemoglobin test confirmed that she now had this condition too.

She said she gained 33 pounds in the last few years and she had high blood pressure. She also reported experiencing low blood glucose, headaches, cramping and yellow, foul smelling stools six to eight times daily. Her feet swelled so much she had difficulty walking.

To try to lose weight Clara ate only 900 calories a day which included high amounts of vegetable fat and too little protein. For breakfast she ate a piece of fruit, sometimes, yogurt, and drank four to five cups of coffee. She knew she could not consume alcohol or smoke tobacco.

The pancreas has several jobs that impact on cells in various parts of the body. Among them, pancreatic cells produce insulin, enzymes to digest food, and bicarbonate, an alkaline substance that neutralizes the acid from the stomach as it enters the top part of the small intestine.

I asked myself several questions about Clara's situation. Could the inability of her pancreas to produce enzymes to digest food have contributed to both her malnourishment and the pneumonia in the earlier years? Was the liver being forced to convert lean tissue cells to glucose? Could malnourishment be the reason her feet were swelling? Could malnourishment contribute to her high blood pressure and gain in weight?

Because Clara's stools were yellow and foul smelling, I suspected she was gluten-sensitive. After she began a 2000-calorie three-meal-a-day regimen without coffee, vegetable fat, or gluten, the abdominal cramps stopped, her stools became firm and normal in color and frequency and she had more energy. After introducing and removing both the wheat and vegetable oil and recording in a diary the reactions, vegetable oil, not the wheat, was identified as the culprit. The undigested oil irritated the intestinal tract cells, preventing the production of the gluten enzyme.

She developed diabetes because her pancreas no longer could produce insulin. Clara eliminated substances that could raise her blood glucose quickly: sugar, vitamin supplements, and caffeine. Coffee is her favorite beverage. She could substitute decaffeinated coffee but it too releases oil from its grounds when heated. She was introduced to "Toddy Coffee" which doesn't release oil (See Chapter Notes).

Clara has improved her health by following a computerized meal plan with enough nutrients and calories to support her lean tissue cells and by eliminating the offending substances. The evidence: blood glucose leveled off at the normal range, her high triglycerides, cholesterol and blood pressure have dropped to normal. She has lost 16 pounds of fat and increased her lean tissue weight all because her body is digesting and absorbing calories and nutrients. She is a happy camper.

Knowing which enzymes are missing means meals can be designed to reduce stress on the digestive system. Unlike vegetable fat, butter fat is already digested when it reaches the small intestine and requires little if any of the enzyme which digest fat from the pancreas or bile from the gallbladder. In fact, a person with gallbladder disease may benefit from consuming butter and animal fats instead of vegetable fats. But whenever it is suggested that people substitute butter for vegetable oil, the question of cholesterol comes up. However, cholesterol is a completely different issue.

At age 47, Betsy had high blood cholesterol. Following the American Heart Association guidelines, she had switched from eating butter to margarine. But then she began experiencing cramping, bloating and flatulence. After two years she sought help. When she returned to butter and eliminated vegetable oils for a week, the cramping disappeared. Additionally, she followed the individualized plan of nutrition *based on her lean tissue weight* that I designed for her. Even though she consumed eggs and butter, her blood cholesterol dropped to normal within three weeks.

The only solution to food intolerances is to identify and then eliminate them since other options are scant. There are few manmade enzymes to replace the thousands produced by the intestinal tract. Medications may be a stop gap solution. Many have side effects, especially with prolonged use. Additionally, some may decrease the absorption of certain vitamins and minerals, making the body lose more lean tissue cells. Drug manufacturers acknowledge these problems: facts are listed in the *Physician's Desk Reference,* a guide to medications, their use, ingredients and adverse reactions.

Sally claimed she had endured diarrhea every day for 25 years. She told me that the medication she was taking did not control it and her doctor could not find the source of the irritation. She said that for 20 to 25 years she had been ingesting a stress formula vitamin pill, 500 milligrams of vitamin C and, for most of that time, 400 International Units of vitamin E to control leg cramps.

I suggested that perhaps the large quantities of vitamins she was consuming were creating a constant irritation in her intestinal tract. After she eliminated the vitamin supplements and vegetable fat and began drinking milk with reduced lactose, Sally's diarrhea stopped. She no longer needed the medication. Months later, she and her husband took a trip to Hawaii for their 50th wedding anniversary. She said it was the first trip they had made in 25 years because she had been tied to the house with its plumbing.

Sally later re-added peanut butter to her diet. With the development of leg cramps, she also added the vitamin E supplements. The diarrhea returned. This convinced her that her body could not process the vegetable fats or the peanuts and that the supplement vitamin E triggered her intestinal tract problems.

Diverticula-Bumps Along the Smooth Digestive Tract

Another problem related to the lack of enzymes is the development of diverticula. Diverticula are areas that form a sac or pouch that bump out through a weak point anywhere along the long tube of the intestinal tract. Weak points occur from irritation or from loss of cells which are recruted for glucose.

Diverticula is fairly common among Americans. In those over the age of 40, it affects more than one-third of the population and, in those over 60, two thirds of the population, making age a factor.

Wherever these diverticula develop, they interfere with the digestion causing a break down of lean tissue and the immune system. Diverticula can erupt into inflammation and infection. The symptoms can be frequent urination, urinary tract or bladder infections, severe cramps, fever and nausea. If the sacs perforate the thin mucous membrane of the thin intestinal tract, an ulcer may develop and may bleed causing pain and anemia.

If the sacs hang on the walls of the large intestine, there may be spasms of diarrhea and constipation causing damage, infection and abcesses. It may be necessary to take an antibiotic to kill off the infection but antibiotics are known irritants. Abscesses may require surgery.

As bad as this sounds, there is hope. By following the "Safe Diet" (See Appendix B) the mucous membranes can recover. The next step is to identify the offending substances and eliminate them from the diet (See Chapter Notes). The longer a person goes without a relapse, the more they can be lulled into thinking that the diverticula have gone away. Then they may slip back into their old habits. Diverticula can be kept under control, but given irritants, diverticulitis, a condition which develops when the diverticula are inflamed, can return.

Solving Other Intestinal Problems
Heartburn And Hiatus Hernia

ENZYMES and acid are produced in the stomach. Both prepare the food for digestion further along the tract. The acid is important. It destroys bacteria that enter through the mouth and nose. It prepares iron, calcium, zinc, potassium and magnesium for absorption in the intestinal tract. The acid environment is just what the enzymes need to digest protein and butter fat. But the stomach is not destroyed. It is beautifully designed to protect itself against the enzymes and the half gallon of very strong hydrochloric acid a day which it produces each day. It is protected by a very thick visco-elastic mucous lining. The stomach even provides protection against acid leakage into other areas. It has a door or sphincter valve—at the stop as well as at the bottom (See Chapter Notes).

But if these beautifully-designed muscular valves become weakened, become spastic, the acid and the enzymes flow through them more freely. Neither the esophagus or the duodenum have the very thick visco-mucous to protect them against the acid and enzymes. When they flow into the esophagus they create reflux, heartburn, bleeding and/or hiatus hernia, the person can then experience pain. When they flow freely into the duodenum, the result is ulcers or scarring (See Chapter Notes for symptoms). An acid burn is bad enough, but the pepsin enzyme digests any protein in its path—be it in food or the protein in the cells of the esophagus or duodenum. When the cells in the esophagus are affected, the person feels heartburn, but it feels like a heart attack. A physician should be consulted immediately (See Chapter Notes).

Nearly 32 million Americans suffer from chronic heartburn, although 62 percent reported[6] they had never spoken to a doctor. Instead, they may pop antacids. The sale of antacids in 1993 was $1 billion. Antacids may make a person feel better temporarily, but they are not a cure. If people continue to ingest antacids, without identifying the cause, the problem can escalate. The acid can continue to damage the esophagus and the duodenum, leading to bleeding and/or cancer.

You know a person has a serious problem when they buy antacids in bulk, always making sure they have some in their pocket or purse and pop them in their mouth continuously.

One man came to my office. I asked him if he was using any medications. He said "No." His wife told him, "Honey, show her what you carry in your pockets." He pulled out several packages of antacids. He told me he kept them in every one of his suit coats.

Antacids themselves have side effects. In young people, the more antacids that are ingested, the more acid the stomach produces. As the stomach ages, less acid is produced. A stomach with less acid cannot digest specific nutrients-such as protein, iron, folic acid, calcium or vitamin A. The unprepared nutrients enter the small intestine and irritate the mucous membranes.

Jean was another challenge.

Jean believed she was experiencing heartburn. This small thin woman had such a bad case of constipation that it kept her awake every night for five years. She was awakened by excessive gas in her abdomen. It took her hours to massage her abdomen downward to express it. She was bloated nearly every day. Her physician examined her and diagnosed gastro-esophageal reflux and prescribed Zantac and Gaviscon. Her constipation became worse.

Believing that food was the cause of the constipation and gas, Jean ingested a lactase enzyme with milk, a multivitamin supplement, herb and garlic tablets, and drank tea and eliminated cauliflower, beans, spices, and greasy foods. But she failed to have a bowel movement for four to five days; even then she had to use a laxative, Milk of Magnesia.

A computer nutrition analysis showed Jean's food intake was only 1000 calories, was excessively low in fat, carbohydrates, potassium, iron, calcium, and vitamin C.

First she eliminated the Gaviscon and Zantac, the vitamins, and, on my advice, added enough calories and nutrients to adequately support her lean tissue cells. Still, she was constipated. She acknowledged that she had never established a regular bowel habit. I suggested a routine that resulted in bowel regularity within two weeks (See Chapter Notes). Since then, she has slept through the night with little or no gas or bloating and is not constipated. However, when she did not have a bowel movement for a few days, the reflux returned. The large amount of feces in her colon were likely pushing against her stomach, forcing the acid to back up into her esophagus.

As is evident from this case, there can be several causes of heartburn, hiatus hernia and reflux (See Chapter Notes). A hiatus hernia is a condition in which the stomach intrudes into the esophagus. The valve at the top of the stomach is too weak to hold it back.

Because Jean was a Muslim, she had to bow down several times a day, which allowed the stomach to push against the weak valve and force it open. For a person with heartburn, hiatus hernia or reflux, there are some simple measures which allow the valves to heal (See Chapter Notes).

Ulcers: Holes in the Fuel Tank

The valve at the top of the stomach and the valve at the bottom can relax and become weak over time by the constant use of caffeine, alcohol, smoking, fried foods, chewing or sucking on peppermint candy or gum.

A weak valve at the bottom of the stomach allows acid and the pepsin enzyme to flow too freely into the duodenum. Normally, the duodenum is kept at an almost neutral pH by bicarbonate released by the pancreas. But the amount of acid flowing into the duodenum can overwhelm the amount of bicarbonate that the pancreas produces. The duodenum also does not have a very thick protective mucous membrane, so the acid and the pepsin enzyme burn the tissue resulting in an ulcer.

For the one in ten people in the United States who have ulcers, this is an exciting time. Recently, it was discovered that a bacteria can live where no one ever thought bacteria could live—in an acid stomach and cause an ulcer.

The bacteria, helicobacter pylori (H. pylori) can take up residence in the duodenum and stomach and live there for 20 or more years gradually doing damage. The presence of the bacteria in the stomach triggers the immune system to release antibodies which create gastritis. The gastritis prevents the enzymes from digesting the food. The food enters the small intestine unprepared for the next step in digestion. If the gastritis is not corrected, gastric carcinoma can develop in about 16 to 24 years.

The antibodies cannot reach the bacteria because it hides in the folds of the mucous membrane. The bacteria freely tunnels through the protective mucous layers of the stomach lining and the duodenum, exposing the unprotected parts to the stomach acid and the pepsin enzyme, eventually producing an ulcer. Early symptoms are belching, bloating and a burning sensation in the area of the breastbone or upper part of the abdomen.

The location of the ulcer, whether in the stomach or duodenum, determines whether the person experiences pain, hemorrhage, and/or lean tissue weight loss. If the ulcer is near a blood vessel, the person can slowly bleed to death. Surgery was and may be the only lifesaving solution for a bleeding ulcer. But surgery does not cure it. A combination of antibiotics and antacids will kill the bacteria about two weeks but the bacteria may return unless the person changes their old habits.

Formerly it was believed that ulcers were caused by the excess acid in the stomach. It was thought the excess acid was brought on by stress, type A personality, dieting, smoking, and alcohol. Perhaps this kind of lifestyle could promote a poorly-nourished body which is unable to resist bacteria entering the stomach through the mouth via food, water or dirty hands. But a healthy body can resist it. A body which is not strong enough to fight it off, can allow H. pylori, a bacteria from human waste, to take up residence. H. pylori prefers the acid environment of the stomach and the duodenum (A healthy body can resist the bacteria).

To be healthy, an intestinal tract, immune system, and valves need enough calories and nutrients which include vitamin A and fat. The vitamin A stimulates the secretion of mucus in the stomach lining and it keeps it healthy and thick. Are people who follow a low-fat diet more at risk for ulcers, diarrhea, or other intestinal track problems such as constipation? Time will tell.

Constipation: The Sluggish Intestinal Track

The intestinal tract is rhythmic like the rest of the body, and is guided by the brain. The brain is like an orchestra leader who directs actions in the body and sets the rhythmic beats of the heart, the rhythmic breathing of the lungs, the rhythmic swallowing of saliva, the rhythmic blinking of the eye, to name a few. Bowel movements, too, are part of this rhythm.

As far as the rhythm of the meals are concerned, when five hours elapse, the hypothalamus triggers the hunger signal. This rhythmic timing has been recognized by many institutions for decades. A regular time is set aside for lunch. How many people ignore the signal and skip lunch? How many people eat meals out of sync with the rhythm of their bodies and eat erratically or eat constantly?

The colon adapts to the rhythm of the body. If the person has an erratic lifestyle, the colon will be erratic too. The colon has muscles which have a rippling rhythmic movement to carry the waste products along. Hormones respond to a rhythm and trigger the muscles to move the waste products out once or twice a day. People may notice that their bowels are irregular when they travel, when they undergo surgery, are in an accident, are ill or have an infection. In fact, constipation may be one of the first signs of the onset of a disease or infection and this is when people should check with their physician. Usually once the disease or infection has been treated and the body has recovered, the constipation resolves itself.

Certain foods you eat, changes in your water or beverages, or certain medications can affect the hormones which control the bowels (See Chapter Notes). Water with iron or calcium deposits may produce either diarrhea or constipation. If it does, you can replace it with reverse osmosis or distilled water.

The colon or large intestine is about six feet long and connects the small intestine with the rectum and anus. It is here that the waste products from the food mass are stored until excreted and returned to the blood along with some mineral, leaving drier feces behind. The bacteria create significant amounts of vitamin K and biotin.

Constipation means the bowels do not move in several days. You experience bloating, pain, gas and hard stools as more water is extracted. Pressure from straining at the stool can lead to a weakening of the intestinal tract walls which in turn can contribute to diverticulosis. Perhaps your brain learned early in life, as at elementary school, to ignore the signal to have a bowel movement. But your brain can be programmed.

You may not want to take the time to retrain your brain but, it is just as important to rid your body of its waste products on a rhythmic schedule, as it is to eat on a rhythmic schedule.

If you use laxatives, the laxatives make the brain and the messages it sends to the bowels sluggish. Constipation must be a growing problem. In 1985, the sales of laxatives were $400 million and in 1991, they were $850 million (See Box 25). Perhaps the people taking laxatives lack rhythm in their everyday life.

If you want to correct or prevent constipation, you can eat upon awaking and then eat rhythmically every five hours after that (See Chapter Notes). Consuming meals in a combination of all six food groups in a pleasant setting can do wonders for the intestinal tract (See Meal Plan in Appendix).

Irritable Bowel, Ulcerative Colitis and Crohn's Disease.

People who have unusually active colons, may have Irritable Bowel Syndrome (IBS). The activity is often triggered by the very act of eating, by stress, and by certain foods, medications, and toxins (See Chapter Notes). Perhaps the person is upset, which of course affects the brain. The brain keeps sending signals for the bowels to move many times a day.

Diarrhea which continues or comes and goes intermittently is one of the first signs of trouble in the intestinal tract. If people wait too long to seek help, they place their bodies in jeopardy. Because each time they have diarrhea, the intestinal tract is irritated and not digesting food. The food travels through too fast for the enzymes to break it down. The body is denied its sources of energy and nutrients. People become dehydrated and malnourished. Their immune system eventually weakens. Their energy is low and their appetite wanes. Adults lose lean tissue weight. Children lose weight and, potentially, height. IBS must be treated because it can develop into ulcerative colitis or Crohn's Disease, two diseases which are difficult to control. Waiting can mean surgery and the surgery may be risky. For Crohn's Disease, the signs are a mild pain in the abdomen and diarrhea. One of the causes of Crohn's disease, according to research, is a larger consumption of sugar and refined carbohydrates than the general population. Calories they may have, but they lack most of the 60 nutrients needed to keep cells healthy.

For ulcerative colitis, the signs are bowel movements that seem imminent but instead only result in gas, water, blood and pus. These signs indicate that the mucous membrane lining of the colon has been perforated, which can result in hemorrhaging and infection.

Treatment of either condition by a physician, and the use of the "Safe Diet" may restore some of the mucous membrane. Learning some relaxation techniques and establishing a rhythmic routine each day may be helpful (See Chapter Notes).

A student in one of my college nutrition classes had Crohn's Disease. She was hospitalized nearly every month, causing her to miss her college classes and drop out for the fall semester. She had several surgeries and used many medications. When she returned the second semester, she chose to follow my "Safe Diet." She baked her own bread, shopped for and prepared her own meals from "scratch," and did not eat in restaurants. With this regime she was able to free herself from complications and to finish the semester. Her attitude improved, she had more self-confidence, her skin had more color and firmness. She also was able to reduce medications. She said "I feel for the first time in years that I have control over my health."

Prevention is the key to preserving the intestinal tract and the health of the body. If the intestinal tract sounds an alarm consult your physician and set aside time to identify the cause or causes by keeping a journal or diary and eliminating the offending substances. The body should be fed real foods with just the right amount of calories and nutrients to support lean tissue. A routine should be established every day for eating meals every five hours, moving the bowels, exercising for 30 minutes, drinking eight to ten glasses of water, sleeping eight hours, relaxing with friends, family and enjoying life. Whether or not one experiences a problem with the intestinal tract, such a regime may be a life saver. And it can also save health dollars. Remember, the intestinal tract is the gateway to the rest of the body.

Chapter Notes:

1: Fruits often reported in the literature as producing gas and diarrhea are bananas, pears, citrus, melons, apples and apple skins. Vegetables reported are broccoli, cauliflower, cabbage, Brussels sprouts, rutabagas, soybeans, turnips, dried beans and peas, onions, garlic, green and red peppers, hot peppers sauerkraut, cucumbers, tomatoes, and radishes. Some people also report problems with tomatoes, vinegars, carbonated beverages, chocolate, tea, coffee, or sugar substitutes and spices (like pepper, cinnamon, ginger, cardamon, chili, mustard, nutmeg; mace, allspice, curry, etc.) Herbs are not a problem unless they are dry. Herbs include parsley, basil, oregano, marjoram, tarragon, sage, etc. Additives, pesticides, herbicides, hormones, or antibiotics added to the food can result in an intestinal upset. Using a diary to record daily food intake and other substances can help identify the culprit.

2: An adult's intestinal tract is a food processor that is 25 to 30 feet long. Food enters the mouth and in seven seconds is ground up by the teeth, swallowed and pushed by muscles down the esophagus through a muscle into the stomach. There it stays for two to five hours and is mixed with acid and liquid. Carbohydrates leave first, followed by protein and then fat. They are pushed through another muscle to the duodenum at the beginning of the small intestine. As the food moves along this assembly line, it takes three hours to be digested by enzymes and chemicals and absorbed. The food mass empties into the colon where water is removed and it is compacted into semi-solid waste. It could remain here for several days before it is excreted. The process takes about 36 to 72 hours. How well this processing plant works is critical to one's health. It also depends on the kinds of foods and beverages, their combinations, the amount, the timing, the environment and lack of interference from offending substances.

3: Single molecules are vitamins, minerals, oxygen, water, glucose from carbohydrate, amino acids from protein, and fatty acids from fat. As mucous cells and enzymes complete their work of breaking the food down, they slough off and are rebuilt. This turnover takes approximately 48 hours.

4: Toxins can be any of the offending substances such as perfumes, underarm deodorant, chemicals such as pesticides, herbicides, cleaning solutions, nail polish or remover, cosmetics, and soap. Sorbitol as well as mannitol, an ingredient in chewing gum, can result in diarrhea. Caffeine is a stimulant that makes the muscles of the colon move.

5: Offending substances; medications especially antibiotics and laxatives, drugs, toxins, vitamin supplements in large doses, food or condiments, disease, infections, polluted water, uncooked meat, infestations, looped intestine, diseased. Inhaled substances that enter the blood and touch the intestinal tract cells. Smoking irritates the gastric membrane and thus sets up pre cancerous conditions in the stomach and esophagus.

6: Hard cheeses are colby, mozzarella, cheddar, Monterey Jack, muenster, parmesan, romano, provolone, and Swiss.

7: Foods with lactose: Liquid and dry milk, cottage cheese, yogurt, cream, sour cream, ice cream, processed cheese, the additive whey, and dry beans such as kidney, lima split, navy, and pinto.

8: Whey contains lactose and is an ingredient in processed cheeses, soft cheeses such as brie, camembert, limburger and cottage cheese. It is present naturally in ice cream, ice milk, sherbet, and uncultured yogurt-frozen or flavored.

9: Lactose is found in such unsuspecting products as medications, weight reduction formulas, iced tea mixes, instant potatoes, instant cereals, wines, and caramel candies, dairy desserts, chocolate cake, orange drink, glaze on bread, and food bars. It also can be injected into ham.

10: Foods that contain gluten are: wheat, rye, barley, oats. Additives that contain gluten are called "starch derivative protein," "vegetable protein." The enzyme that is commercially made to digest lactose in milk is cultured on wheat. Fillers for pills and vitamins have wheat starch. A great deal of material may be obtained on-line. Type in Celiac LISTSERV, Fact Sheet.

11: Blood tests can reveal sprue or celiac disease. Blood glucose is low. Hemoglobin is low from the loss of red blood cells. Creatinine and protein are low indicating starvation and loss of lean tissue. In addition, the ankles are swollen with water (edema). Muscles will spasm (called tetany) from low absorption of Vitamin D, calcium and magnesium. Loss of these nutrients means bone cells are lost too.

12: Toddy coffee is brewed overnight in cold water and filtered the next morning. The coffee will remain fresh for two or three weeks provided it is stored in the refrigerator. Boiling water is added to make a cup of hot or cold coffee.

13: The stomach protects the esophagus and duodenum tubes by having "doors"—one at the top, the other at the bottom. The top "door" is the cardiac or lower esophageal sphincter (LES). It allows food to pass into the stomach and then snaps shut to prevent the acid from backing up into the esophagus. The bottom "door" is the pyloric sphincter and prevents the acid from flowing freely into the duodenum. The sphincter allows only small amounts of food to pass into the duodenum before it snaps shut. The acid contents that flow from the stomach are immediately neutralized by bicarbonate, a neutralizing agent from the pancreas. People sometimes take "bicarbonate of soda" to suppress the acid in their stomach. Not a good idea.

14: Symptoms of heartburn or esophageal reflux are a painful burning sensation in the center of the chest, discomfort after eating spicy foods, difficulty in swallowing, an acid or bitter taste in the mouth.

15: Symptoms of a heart attack: chest pains, nausea, vomiting, weakness, breathlessness, fainting, or sweating. A physician must be consulted immediately.

16: To establish a bowel habit is to essentially train the brain. The routine works best if the person sets aside a half hour after breakfast each morning. Then he or she inserts in the rectum a glycerine suppository which is composed of wax. This laxative only affects the rectum, not the whole intestinal tract. The brain take about 15 minutes to register that it needs to stimulate the nerves to move the bowels. The procedure should be repeated each morning until the suppository is no longer needed, probably about 2 weeks. Laxatives which are taken by mouth make the brain lazy and do not help establish a regular bowel habit. Laxatives also can change the electrolytes, resulting in serious medical problems.

17: Drugs that can relax the sphincters and produce reflux include Theophylline, calcium channel blockers, hormones like estrogen, progesterone, aspirin, indomethacin, (an anti-arthritic drug), tricyclic antidepressants, beta and alpha adrenergic antagonists, diazepam, and meperidine. Other substances are, fried foods, vitamin supplements especially vitamin C and niacin, (ascorbic acid and nicotinic acid), alcohol, chocolate, caffeine and nicotine.

Steps to prevent heartburn, reflux and hiatus hernia:

- Avoid spicy, acidic and tomato based foods such as fruit juice, pizza, jalapeno peppers, lemons, limes, oranges, and grapefruit.
- Avoid fatty foods or anything that is fried.
- Alcohol, caffeine, chocolate relax the sphincter muscles and allow stomach acid to pass through.
- Avoid carbonated beverages. Belching, the swallowing of air, can bring stomach acid up through the cardiac sphincter into the esophagus.
- Try to keep weight normal. Overweight increases pressure in the abdominal area which can push the stomach into the esophagus.

Eat small amounts of foods slowly at mealtime. Large meals distend the stomach which push up against the esophagus. Eat meals 3 to 4 hours before lying down. Sit or stand upright for an hour after eating. Avoid bedtime snacks.

Sip water or liquid rather than drinking it throughout the meal and make it luke-warm. Cool hot foods slightly and warm ice cold foods a little.

Wait an hour before exercising after a meal. Instead of running, walk about 30 to 40 minutes about three times a week. Jumping up and down can force the sphincter muscle open.

Physically, gravity can keep the acid down in the stomach. The best way to sleep is on a slant. Pillows can be placed under the mattress but not under the head. Or cement blocks can be placed under the legs of the headboard.

Bending over can open the sphincter and allow acid to flow into the esophagus. Sitting erect is better than being hunched over, and stooping with bent knees to pick something up is better than bending over.

Quit smoking because nicotine relaxes the pyloric sphincter muscles.

When swallowing a pill, whether it is a medication or a vitamin supplement, it is better to stand, sip a little water, then pop the pill into the mouth and follow it with a whole glass of water. Remain standing for another 90 seconds. Otherwise, the pill may not travel all the way to the stomach and may dissolve in the esophagus and injure cells. Acid pills, like vitamin C may dissolve on the way through the esophagus and can burn the stomach lining.

Medications which seem to damage the esophagus are: tetracycline, doxcycline, quinidine, slow release potassium chloride, iron salts, and nonsteroidal anti-inflammatory drugs.

Drink at least 8 glasses of water every day, preferably bottled.

A full stomach, tight belts, girdles, and panty hose can force the cardiac sphincter open. Wearing loose clothing will not be restrictive.

Spasms of the sphincter can be caused by swallowing large mouthfuls of food, or chunks of meat, raw fruits, and vegetables, nuts, peanut or sesame or soy butters. But well-cooked food which is soft, moist, chopped and prepared without spices most likely will not.

18: Preventing the invasion of H. pylori: Washing hands before handling or consuming food is probably the best deterrent. H. pylori can establish itself in the plaque of the teeth but may not if the teeth are professionally cleaned twice a year. To fight off the bacteria, the immune system can be strengthened and the mucous membranes in the intestinal tract can be rebuilt with enough calories and nutrients to support the lean tissue cells. However, an alcohol drink or two every evening before dinner can cancel out the vitamin A consumed in the meal. Vitamin A is necessary to build up the immune system and mucous mem-branes. The liver stores vitamin A but cannot while it's detoxifying the alcohol.

19: Causes of constipation: Adapted from National Digestive Diseases Information Clearinghouse, A service of the National Institute of Diabetes and Digestive and Kidney Diseases, National Institutes of Health, Washington, DC

- Poor diet and too little water
- Irritable Bowel Syndrome or spastic colon
- Bowel habits
- Laxative Abuse-insensitive intestinal tract
- Travel-changes in lifestyle, routine, diet and water
- Hormonal disturbances-like hypothyroidism
- Pregnancy-changes in the hormones and physical pressure on the abdomen from the fetus
- Fissures and hemorrhoids
- Diseases including mental illnesses
- Vomiting and diarrhea
- Mechanical compression
- Nerve damage

- Medications
- Convenience foods-no bulk or fiber
- Emotions
- Lack of exercise

I would add lack of rhythm in the daily life.

20: The medications that can produce constipation are: progestin hormone (a type of estrogen) which slows the muscles pushing the food mass through the intestinal tract. It also can cause straining at the stool and irritation of the veins in the anal region resulting in hemorrhoids. Other medications that can cause constipation are: codeine-containing pain relievers, antidepressants and aluminum containing antacids.

21: The problem with laxatives: The brain can become too dependent on laxatives. Laxatives in general can prevent the absorption of fat soluble vitamins and cause the loss of lean tissue. Laxatives contain phosphorus which can deplete the bone of calcium and can change the mineral balance in the blood resulting in heart arrhythmias.

Mineral oil coats the entire lining of the intestinal tract thus preventing the absorption of fat soluble vitamins and other nutrients.

Castor oil prevents the colon wall from absorbing water which can result in dehydration. With long term use castor oil can damage the cells of the colon and intensify constipation between doses.

Milk of Magnesia taken over a period of time can produce slurring of speech, unsteadiness, lethargy, profuse sweating, abnormal heart rhythms, and drowsiness.

Recommendations for preventing constipation:

- Consult with a physician if bowels change in regularity, content or color for several days.
- Consume about 2000-2400 calories with all 60 nutrients divided into three meals five hours apart (See meal plans).
- Include fiber in the meals such as whole fruits instead of juices (three a day), whole vegetables (two to three a day), eight servings from the starch group like potatoes (with their skins), whole grain breads and cereals, legumes, and corn, brown rice, bran cereals, whole wheat pasta, etc. Incorporate one of these foods every day into the menu: watermelon, parsley, garlic, cantaloupe or honeydew melon, or coriander (a spice).
- In the meals, include two to three teaspoons of fat, in the form of oil (not margarine or hydrogenated fats) or butter. Also, include foods with vitamin A such as eggs, butter, cheese, and milk.
- Use lactose reduced milks or substitute hard cheeses or yogurt with active culture.
- Sip two glasses of water with each meal and one between meals. When traveling, carry water from home or buy reverse osmosis or distilled water.
- Maintain a regular daily bowel habit. Some people drink a glass of warm lemon water before breakfast to stimulate the colon to move.
- Keep medications to a minimum and change or reduce medications that can cause constipation. Consult with a physician before ingesting over the counter medications or eliminate them, especially, antacids, cold syrups, laxatives.

- Allow eight hours for sleep.
- Wear loose clothing.
- Exercise for 30 to 40 minutes each day-preferably walking, swimming or bicycling.

22: A regime to stop the diarrhea. If laxatives have been used, they should be discontinued. On day one, eliminate fat. or add medium chain triglycerides (MCT oil), white chicken or turkey, baked potato or plain rice, hot cereal (grits or cream of rice) (no milk) scraped apple, gelatin, and plenty of distilled water. On the second day add baby food vegetables and fruits and baked or broiled lean meat. If there is no diarrhea, add on the third day a slice of white toast. After day four the medium chain triglycerides can be replaced with butter. MCT oil can be purchased through the pharmacist. Use one to two teaspoons at each meal. Other recommendations to make the intestinal tract healthy is to eliminate the offending substances. Salt and herbs can make the dishes more tasty. Tight belts and panty hose can make the abdomen uncomfortable. Elevate the feet for one half hour daily and delay exercise for a few weeks.

CHAPTER 4

Feed Your Liver
And Control Your Cholesterol

HIGH blood cholesterol has been identified as one factor in the development of heart disease and one that people can control. What do you think are the causes of high blood cholesterol? (See Chapter Notes for answers).

High blood cholesterol may be the result of: (True or False)

- Too much fat?
- Too much cholesterol?
- Too much unsaturated fat ?
- Too few calories?
- Too little fat?
- Hydrogenated fat?
- Fried fats?
- Megadoses of vitamin C?
- Too much sugar?
- Too much alcohol?
- Too much zinc?
- Too much caffeine?
- Excess estrogen?
- Skipping meals?
- Smoking cigarettes or cigars?
- Stress?
- Too much body fat?
- Underactive thyroid?
- Disease of kidney, intestinal tract or liver?
- No aerobic exercise?
- Pregnancy?

A History of Blood Cholesterol

It all dates to the 1950's when The American Heart Association found scientific evidence proving cholesterol collects in blood vessels. Eventually, blood vessels become blocked resulting in a heart attack. During a heart attack body cells will die unless blood flow with its nourishment is restored immediately.

Today heart disease is the leading medical problem in the United States, causing 1.5 million heart attacks and 500,000 premature deaths per year. An estimated 6 million Americans have a history of heart attacks and/or angina pectoris before age 65 (See Chapter Notes).

The American Heart Association's (AHA) and The National Cholesterol Education Program's goal is to reduce heart disease by educating the public and the medical profession about the dangers of heart disease. The AHA found in the 1950's that Americans were consuming over 30 percent of their diet in fat and that too much dietary fat was a factor in high blood cholesterol. They recommended that dietary fat intake be reduced to 30 percent, saturated fat to 10 percent of the calories and dietary cholesterol to 300 mg.

However, these are not the *only* factors that will lead to high blood cholesterol, of which the most important one is to feed the body enough calories and nutrients to keep the liver healthy. This is an obvious omission which leaves a large gap in past research. To understand what those factors are is to understand how the liver works to prevent disease.

The liver is one of the body's unsung heroes. It is a very large manufacturing plant with an exclusive contract to supply the body's 75 trillion cells with nutritional products. When the liver receives its share of glucose and nutrients, it produces and excretes cholesterol, stores glucose and nutrients, protects body cells from toxins, and provides materials to rebuild them. This manufacturing plant never closes, never takes a vacation, and is available to its customers, the body cells, 24 hours a day, seven days a week.

To do all this work, the liver cells use about 300 calories or 75 grams of glucose a day. Even though liver cells have a crucial role in the body's functions and produce glucose, they are not first in line for its use. As explained in Chapter 2, the first to use glucose are the brain, nerves and red blood cells. These require 750 calories or 180 grams per day.

As you again look at the questions at the beginning of the chapter, keep in mind that the liver, like the rest of the body, needs energy from food. Several questions deal with fat so let's first define how much is too little in dietary fat, saturated fat, and dietary cholesterol.

Restrict Your Calories and Increase Your Stress

Yes, high blood cholesterol is a problem. But it is difficult for people to translate the recommended fat percentages into meals. You have been told for years to LOWER YOUR FAT INTAKE. And not knowing whether you are consuming too much, you may believe dietary fat is not necessary or that your body will use body fat in its place. With this in mind, you may overly restrict your intake of dietary fat. With less fat you are probably consuming less calories and may lose weight (lean tissue weight). Your blood cholesterol may drop, but often it will rise again, or it may not drop at all and even continue rising. What went wrong? You did what was recommended. It must be the genes. Better take medication . . . But wait a minute. Did anyone mention calories or that the lack thereof can cause heart disease, stress and high blood cholesterol?

Erma was an, underweight woman in her 70's who had high blood cholesterol. When she came to see me, she had so little energy she could barely move. Her face was pinched and she had a furrowed brow (often a sign of malnutrition). Although she had been taking a cholesterol-reducing medication, her blood cholesterol level remained high even though she had also reduced her dietary fat intake. When I analyzed her food intake, it was down to 700 calories a day. She had not been told to replace the fat calories with carbohydrates. She had difficulty consuming more food, but with encouragement, she was able to eat 1800 calories with 25 percent fat and an increase in starch. She did gain five pounds—but measurements revealed it was all in lean tissue! Her energy improved and the *stress* signs left her face. In three months, her blood cholesterol levels dropped to normal.

Usually, stress is defined as too many family or job hassles and not enough time or energy to solve them. Well-known causes of stress include death of a loved one, money problems, poor health, divorce, loss of job, etc. The more stress the body has, the harder the liver cells must work, and therefore the greater the health problems (See Chapter Notes for other stresses on the liver). But the greatest stress you can put on your body is to consume too few calories.

Jerry was a prosecuting attorney who worked ten or more hours daily. He bicycled weekends, was not overweight, but had stress lines in his face. He said he ate no breakfast, claimed he had no time for lunch, and reported he didn't eat dinner many evenings until eight o'clock. His cholesterol level was high. His dinner habits didn't change, but he added breakfast (that included an egg), lunch and an afternoon snack each day. After ten days he had a blood test. His cholesterol level was normal and the stress lines were gone. It was hard to believe that his cholesterol level could drop that much in 10 days.

When liver cells do not receive enough glucose (energy) and nutrients from food, they can function erratically and eventually falter resulting in the whole body being affected—one thing leading to another just like dominos (See Chapter Notes for more information on the liver).

Reducing stress and blood cholesterol may be as simple as consuming 2000 calories a day for women and 2400 for men, distributed over three meals and a snack (See Meal Plans in Appendix). Researchers say that consuming the bulk of one's calories early in the day and allowing plenty of time before consuming more should improve how cells handle fat, produce insulin, and control the fluidity of the blood—all important factors in coronary health. Dr. Renata Cifkova, a researcher at Memorial University of Newfoundland, reported that blood platelets are more apt to clump together when a person skips breakfast.[7] Taking that a step further, wouldn't blood be thicker when other meals are skipped? When blood platelets clump together, they reduce the blood flow in the arteries; when the body is under stress from the lack of calories and nutrients, the blood thickens. Everything in the blood is more concentrated, including the blood fats.

Researchers have studied the French because they wondered why the French have a lower heart disease rate than Americans. The French eat butter, cream, high fat meals and smoke cigarettes. Is it because they consume more red wine and fresh vegetables? Or is it because they eat 60 percent of their calories before two p.m., whereas Americans eat less than 40 percent. The French are wiser. Their ritual is to eat three meals a day. They eat breakfast, eat their main meal at noon and are more active before they eat again five hours later. Many Americans skip breakfast and often lunch. They are less active and snack every few hours. What office does not have treats on the desk and coffee and soda pop machines in the lounge? How does some or all of this lifestyle affect the cells that use fat and produce insulin and triglycerides?

Carolyn, a grandmother, had an extremely high blood cholesterol reading. She came to see me with a contorted face and said, "I'm going to die." She believed she was following a low-fat and low-cholesterol diet to keep her blood cholesterol normal. But she skipped either breakfast or lunch, depending on her hectic schedule. She swam in her indoor pool regularly. I suggested she eat three times daily with enough calories and nutrients to support her lean tissue. As a result her cholesterol level dropped to almost normal in three weeks without medication. She gloatingly told her friends that it dropped even though she ate an egg each morning and butter instead of margarine. Over the next three months, she lost 12 more pounds of fat. A year later, she became concerned that although her cholesterol level was below the recommended level, she had regained seven pounds. A review of her eating habits revealed that she had added fruit yogurt and frozen yogurt to her daily diet because "they were low in fat and cholesterol." But they were high in sugar.

Low-Fat or No-Fat Diets

People who overly restrict their fat intake not only are restricting their calories but their body may not have enough dietary fat to stimulate the liver to produce bile a substance which processes cholesterol and excretes it. And without enough fat from food, as distinguished from body fat, the fat soluble vitamins are not absorbed as they pass through the intestinal tract. The person can become malnourished as discussed in chapter two.

Without fat soluble vitamin A, mucous membranes can dry up and the immune system diminish. Without fat soluble vitamin E the LDL part of blood cholesterol can oxidize—resulting in sticky plaques building up in the blood vessels. Sticky plaques can result in heart attacks, blood clots and strokes. The amount of vitamin E the body needs is very small—only 30 I.U. daily. Foods can easily supply this: eggs, nuts, whole grains and oils. But many vitamin manufacturers and physicians suggest that people take this antioxidant in supplement form—400 I.U. daily. Initially it may help, especially if a person has not been consuming foods with vitamin E. But ingesting 400 I.U. is 1300 times more vitamin E than the body can use and can disturb the balance of other nutrients. Taken over a long period of time, the extra vitamin E which is not used can accumulate, be stored and lead to toxicity. When it does, it interferes with the cells' ability to use and absorb other nutrients such as vitamins B12 and K. Without vitamin B12, the person becomes anemic and, without vitamin K, the blood does not clot as readily resulting in bleeding and hemorrhages. Vitamin K is also a fat soluble vitamin and depends on dietary fat to be absorbed from foods.

Vitamin D is the another fat soluble vitamin. Without enough vitamin D, calcium is not absorbed and bones deteriorate. Bone loss is not as detectable as a lingering cold or an ear ache, but it does happen.

Rev Up Your Bile to Reduce Blood Cholesterol

As said before, without enough dietary fat, the liver is not stimulated to produce bile, an important enzyme in reducing and controlling cholesterol levels in the blood. Normally, the liver produces more cholesterol than the cells can pick up and use, but it covers itself by producing bile to carry the excess from the body.

However, without enough bile, cholesterol collects into a thick mucus-like material full of crystals. And suddenly one day a person experiences pain, vomiting, pancreatitis because this biliary sludge is too thick to pass through the narrow opening in the duodenum. Blood cholesterol can rise. These symptoms and signs occur after a person has been following a low fat diet or it happens to a woman who is pregnant, is over 40 and obese and/or taking estrogen. With these conditions, the liver produces more cholesterol and less bile.

Animal Fats Versus Vegetable Fats

Many people equate cholesterol with saturated fat and believe if they reduce their intake of saturated fat, they will be healthier. But will they? The marketability of products with vegetable fat has made saturated fats very unpopular and unprofitable. Vegetable fats have been enhanced with labels of *no cholesterol, cholesterol free, contains no cholesterol, or reduced cholesterol* (See Chapter Notes). These products have sold so well that "total fat intake in the United States has risen through the years, according to S.M. Grundy," a noted medical researcher.[8] Confirming this is a 1994 survey by the United States Department of Agriculture.[9] Five of the top ten sources of fat are hydrogenated with margarine in the number one position, followed by shortening, mayonnaise and salad dressing. Items with saturated fats such as eggs, butter and ice cream are at the bottom.

Does consuming all of this vegetable fat have any impact on blood cholesterol? Fat is fat no matter what the source. Vegetable fats are liquid, contain no cholesterol, and are polyunsaturated. So far this meets the guidelines. However, people want a fat that looks and spreads like butter and fries like lard. Butter and lard are solid because they are naturally saturated with hydrogens. So manufacturers add hydrogens to liquid polyunsaturated vegetable fats and made them solid. Examples are margarine and shortenings which proliferate in the food supply. They are found in cakes, cookies, crackers, bakery products, and shortening used to fry potatoes, doughnuts, chips, battered chicken and seafood, taco shells, etc. But the process of adding hydrogens to the liquid polyunsaturated fats, converts them to trans-fatty acids and destroys linoleic acid. Trans-fatty acids have been found to not only raise LDL, the "bad cholesteral," but lower the HDL, the "good cholesterol." It has not been determined how much trans-fatty acid will raise LDL.

Linoleic acid and linolenic acids are two essential fatty acids in liquid vegetable fats. They are necessary for growth, to prevent skin rashes, to prevent the rise of blood cholesterol, and to prevent the breakdown of the immune system (See Chapter Notes for sources of linoleic and linolenic acids). But when they have been destroyed either by adding hydrogens or by frying, people can develop some serious medical problems. Frying not only destroys linoleic and linolenic acids and vitamin E, it also oxidizes them. And oxidized fats are a factor in the development of heart disease. Of great concern are the low birth-weight babies born to mothers who may not have known that hydrogenated and fried fats and a low-fat diet prevent their babies' growth. Trans-fatty acids do not transfer from the mother to the child, reducing not only the calories but fat and linoleic acid necessary for the normal growth of the fetus.

So much for manipulating unsaturated fats!

Which do you think is better, butter or margarine? Actually, the problem is not so much the kind of fat but the amount. A teaspoon of butter has the same amount of fat as a teaspoon of margarine, I'll take the butter for its taste and nutrients.

Another kind of fat, monounsaturated fat, contains no cholesterol and has a small amount of linoleic and linolenic acid. "Mono" means it is missing only one hydrogen but it is still liquid. Monounsaturated fats are found in peanut, rice, olive and avocado oils. These oils are not usually used for frying but they are used to sauté foods and add flavor. Since these oils can deteriorate fast, they must be refrigerated after they are opened. Some people have misinterpreted the messages they have heard about monounsaturated fats. They have the idea that fats which are monounsaturated are better for them than fats which are saturated or polyunsaturated and they can consume them in larger quantities. One lady told me she was drinking olive oil and rice oil to lower her blood cholesterol.

Eggs Are Not Bad for You

The emphasis to reduce dietary cholesterol has created other misconceptions. For instance, the reputation of eggs has suffered. An egg does have 213 to 289 mg of cholesterol—depending on its size. One egg a day has little effect on blood cholesterol. But often they are the first food to be removed from the breakfast table even though it has never been proven that eggs raise blood cholesterol. Eggs have nutrients that protect the body and lean tissue cells. Eggs contain some fat (5.4 grams), but only two grams are saturated. They have many important virtues. They have *the highest biological protein of any food,* and contain the very nutrients that the liver uses to control blood cholesterol. The amount of cholesterol that is absorbed in the intestinal tract from an egg depends on the meal's fiber content. The best sources of fiber are fresh fruit and vegetables, whole grain bread and brown rice.

Why haven't eggs been taken off the National Cholesterol Education Program's list of foods that raise blood cholesterol, when other foods which contain more were removed in 1988?[10] (The foods removed were shrimp, lobster and clams). Research has shown that these seafoods do not raise blood cholesterol if they are not fried.

Dietary Cholesterol vs. Blood Cholesterol

As you can see from the above information, the basic assumption made 30 years ago that dietary cholesterol will raise blood cholesterol is in trouble. Actually, foods that contain cholesterol have little impact on how much cholesterol the liver will produce. In fact, if you were breast-fed as an infant, your liver learned very early to handle the cholesterol in breast milk. At the other end of the lifeline, if a person is over 70 years of age, high blood cholesterol at this age is not caused by diet nor is medication warranted because high blood cholesterol does not increase morbidity. In fact, cholesterol screening is not recommended by The American College of Physicians, (the nation's largest organization of internists), for young adults, men younger than 35 and women younger than 45 or for anyone over 65 unless they have clear risk factors.[11]

Other problems with reducing or eliminating dietary cholesterol and saturated fat also have been uncovered in the past 30 years. Recent research has found two: one is the threat of cancer, the other, the threat of anemia.

People who consume polyunsaturated fats exclusively or in large quantity have a higher risk for cancer. Polyunsaturated fats thin the cell membranes, allowing the invasion of cancer into any cell. Additionally, hexane and benzene are sometimes used to extract oil from soybeans, corn and seeds. A residue in the oil. Hexane and benzene are gasoline derivatives which, if consumed or inhaled in quantities or often enough, can result in cancer. They also can irritate and injure the mucous membrane cells of the intestinal tract. And if the intestinal tract is irritated on a daily basis for a period of time it can make a person anemic, malnourished and eventually may lead to cancer.

The threat of anemia depends on a person's intake of iron and other red blood cell building nutrients. These nutrients are iron, copper and B12, which are higher in red meats, eggs and egg yolks than other foods. But because of their content of saturated fats, people may have eliminated the very nutrients which can keep them from becoming anemic. If they are anemic, they will notice they are fatigued, confused, have headaches and memory loss. They need to add back into their diet red meats and eggs in moderation and enough calories to support their lean tissue.

The National Cholesterol Education Program and American Heart Association professionals revised their recommendations in 1989.[12] They now suggest that *avoiding* eggs, red meats, butter, cheese, and animal fats is risky. The recommendations *always did state* that one-third of the total fat should be from foods with saturated fat. But this was never widely publicized. Unfortunately, most of the medical profession still recommends and the public still believes that it is healthier to consume polyunsaturated fats such as margarine and oils and eliminate saturated fat.

Saturated fats are allowed, but most people are unsure how much or how to translate that into food. The total grams of fat a day, using a woman as an example and based on the recommended 2000 calories, calculates out to 56 to 66 with 18 to 22 grams from saturated fat (See Chapter Notes). Therefore, every day, a woman can consume three ounces of lean red meat, one egg, three teaspoons of butter and an ounce of cheese as long as she also includes oils which are unsaturated fats. An example of the unsaturated oils is six teaspoons of oil from corn or soy, not fried or hydrogenated, and six teaspoons of olive oil or canola oil. (See meals in Appendix).

Cholesterol Reducing Medications

How many people have a low-fat diet spelled out like this for them? Some people would rather take a pill than to change the habits which led to their high blood cholesterol in the first place. Some believe the cholesterol-reducing medications are a magic bullet. A woman acquaintance said to me, "As long as I take my pill, I do not need to worry about what I eat or drink." She said she was not instructed on a diet, or of changing her lifestyle (smoking) and therefore assumed they were not important. She believed what her doctor told her; the cholesterol-reducing medication would take care of her blood cholesterol.

How motivated would anybody be to change his or her diet or investigate the underlying problem when the medication can miraculously reduce blood cholesterol? Cholesterol-reducing medications, like other medications, have their side effects. Many of them are based on the premise that preventing the absorption of fat will prevent the production of cholesterol. With less absorption of fat, blood cholesterol may or may not drop. But what is more important, they can prevent the absorption of fat-soluble vitamins. As was said earlier, reduced absorption of fat-soluble vitamins can lead to a reduced immune system and malnourishment. Many of the side effects are listed in the Physicians Desk Reference (See Chapter Notes for list of cholesterol reducing medications).[13]

Sometimes people in their zeal to lower blood cholesterol jump from the frying pan into the fire.

Julie, a large-framed woman in her 60's, needed to reduce her cholesterol level and lose weight. Her physician had prescribed a cholesterol-reducing medication. When she came to see me, she had had a cold for four months. But even though she followed the meal plan I provided for her, she could not shake the cold. Her doctor agreed that she could eliminate the medication. The cold symptoms disappeared.

Jocelyn, a thin woman in her 70's, had been following an extremely low-fat diet when she first came to see me ten years ago. Her doctor had prescribed a cholesterol-reducing medication. Every three or four weeks for a year, she took an antibiotic to treat a recurring bladder infection. When she discontinued the cholesterol-reducing medication, increased her fat intake to 25 percent, and added enough calories to support her lean tissue cells, these infections stopped. However, not convinced and scared about having a heart attack, she eventually returned to a low fat diet. Now she has returned with intermittent diarrhea and constipation. And she keeps losing weight.

I have worked with numerous people with diverse symptoms that led me to suspect their cholesterol-reducing medications combined with their low fat diets were causing them to have dry mucous membranes. One person had a cold for four months, followed by hearing problems. Another woman had a vaginal infection for several months. Another had bladder infections intermittently. A computer program was used to analyze their diets. Each of their diets were extremely low in fat—only 6 to 15 grams of fat in a day. In all of these cases, once these people increased their fat intake to between 55 to 60 grams, and were given permission by their physician to discontinue the medication, the symptoms disappeared.

Your goal is to follow a diet which contains the right number of calories and nutrients to support your lean tissue with no less than 25 and not more than 30 percent of the calories in fat. Even with this healthy diet, there can be offenders which can torpedo your attempt at keeping your blood cholesterol low.

Other Offenders and Blood Cholesterol

Other offenders are the lack or or excess of certain nutrients, medications, lack of exercise, sugar, alcohol, caffeine and smoking.

Vitamin C in high doses over (500 mg) can hinder the production of the insulin hormone resulting in a rise in blood glucose, a rise in blood cholesterol and triglycerides, a rise in the formation of kidney stones or oxalate excretion and prevent the absorption of copper. It can interfere with the absorption of vitamin E, resulting in oxidation of LDL and a rise in blood cholesterol.

A 16-year-old male was diagnosed with diabetes when he was 10. He followed an individualized meal plan. As he grew, I adjusted his computerized meal plan to reflect his need for increased calories . . . from 2400 to 5000 daily. But at 17, his blood glucose levels became abnormally high which meant he needed more insulin. His cholesterol had risen and he complained of a new symptom . . . nausea in the morning. A review of his lifestyle revealed he was ingesting 480 milligrams of vitamin C daily from fruit juices and 500 milligrams from a supplement. He had read that the vitamin C prevents colds. When he eliminated the vitamin C supplement and drank water instead of fruit juice, he was able to control his blood glucose levels with less insulin and his blood cholesterol levels dropped to normal.

Large doses of vitamin C can also affect how the cells handle various drugs. For example, the concentration of estrogen, prescribed either for birth control or after menopause, increases. An increase in estrogen can cause high blood cholesterol (See Chapter Notes).

When Eloise reached menopause, her physician prescribed estrogen to "prevent osteoporosis." No one told her to discontinue the large dose (1000 to 2000 mg) of vitamin C that she had been taking faithfully for years "to prevent colds." Two years later she developed breast cancer and high blood cholesterol. She reported that her doctor thought the estrogen was not the cause of cancer but it stimulated it's growth. Neither her physician or she were aware that magadosses of vitamin C can increase the toxicity of estrogen or increase blood cholesterol. In addition, because she gained weight on the estrogen, she reduced her caloric intake to 750 calories a day (calculated by computer analysis). I suggested she eliminate the vitamin C which she did but I could not convince her to increase her calories. Two months later she developed heart arrhythmias and was told by the doctor to reduce her weight. He suggested she follow a 1200 calorie meal plan but again she refused. She did not like my suggestion that she eat more and stopped coming to see me.

Ingesting large doses of vitamin C supplements also can lead to a rise in triglycerides, another blood fat used for energy. Niacin ingested in large doses can also lead to a rise in blood triglycerides, blood glucose and uric acid. Because of this, diabetics and those with gout are warned not to take either vitamin C or niacin in supplement form.

Zinc in supplement form also can raise blood cholesterol. Zinc is necessary every day for about 300 reactions in the body. People may take zinc supplements because they wish to improve their immune system or to slow macular degeneration of the eyes, to ward off colds or to improve their appetite. But large doses of zinc can interfere with the absorption of copper and iron (See Chapter Notes for food sources of zinc).

Certain medications can increase blood cholesterol, particularly if taken on a long term basis (See Chapter Notes). A pharmacist or a physician can recommend alternatives.

Triglycerides

With all the attention paid to blood cholesterol, blood triglycerides have all but been overlooked. Triglycerides and cholesterol are equally important because what affects one affects the other (See Chapter Notes).

A person can be correct in believing that high blood triglycerides *are* caused by too much fat on the body, too much fat in the diet, too many carbohydrates like sugar, too much alcohol and too many calories in the meal. Genetics also can play a part (See Chapter Notes).

Blood triglycerides are fats in the blood. The body always need a certain amount—about 150 mg/dL some of which the cells use as energy. Fat in the blood is different than fat in our food, although both are called triglycerides. Fat in our food has several purposes. It adds taste, smell and a feeling of satisfaction. It slows the progress of food through the intestinal tract so the enzymes have a chance to digest it. It stimulates the liver to produce bile, and it carries fat soluble vitamins through the intestinal tract to the liver. Fat on the body is used as insulation, cushions the organs, and is an alternative fuel to glucose.

After the dietary fats are digested in the intestinal tract to fatty acids, the fatty acids travel to the liver where enzymes are programmed to dismantle and reorganize them into triglycerides. Then they are sent out into the blood stream for certain cells to pick up and use as energy. Some are stored as fat pads to be converted into fatty acids and used by the muscles at a later date. Another source of fatty-acids are excess protein and carbohydrates, especially sugar. Excess fatty acids are converted in the liver to body fat for insulation and cushioning (See Chapter Notes).

If triglycerides accumulate in the blood abnormally, the blood becomes thick and creamy. The thicker blood is more difficult for the heart to pump, raising blood pressure.

High blood triglycerides mean something is amiss with the liver enzymes or the pancreas (See Chapter Notes).

If a person has more than 20 percent body fat, the liver and muscle cells may resist insulin and then glucose molecules tend to accumulate in the blood. The liver then converts them to triglycerides.

Other substances that raise blood triglycerides are sugar, especially because of its fructose content, alcohol, caffeine and some medications (See Chapter Notes). These increase the number of glucose molecules in the blood too fast for the cells to pick them up. So the excess is converted by the liver enzymes to triglycerides.

CHAPTER 4a

More Care and Feeding of the Liver

Subtle Fat Vendors

MR. Young, a 65 year old man, was confused by the messages he received about his diet. He had high blood cholesterol. His wife practically eliminated the fat and cholesterol from his meals making his meal less satisfying. He was hungry all the time. He discovered to his delight that hard candy had no cholesterol and no fat, so he popped hard candy in his mouth all day long. So what if he gained 40 pounds in a year and his blood cholesterol remained high, he was doing what he had been told.

Because of their effect on the liver, alcohol and sugar cause blood glucose to rise and the person feels good for a short period of time. Then blood glucose drops and the person feels the need for another "fix." Sugar and alcohol have a very low satiety level, making them more addictive. With alcohol, the more a person drinks, the less desire he or she has for food. For some people, the same may be true about sugar.

Additionally, sugar and alcohol bring no nutrients to the liver cells' dinner table. But, in order for them to be processed, nutrients are needed. As an example copper, one of these nutrients, is needed to produce alcohol dehydrogenase, an enzyme produced in the liver. Alcohol dehydrogenase breaks down the alcohol into harmless particles which the bile picks up and excretes. Although copper is stored in the liver, when alcohol and sugar replace food, not only is copper depleted from the stores, it is not replenished. When the supply of copper is low or nonexistent, blood cholesterol rises and less alcohol dehydrogenase is produced (See Chapter Notes). The undigested particles of alcohol become harmful. They float around in the blood, damaging cells they touch. If the beta cells in the pancreas are damaged, the person can develop diabetes, either

Type I or II. If the diabetes is not controlled, blood cholesterol and triglycerides can rise.

A person may be told that two alcoholic drinks may improve their blood cholesterol levels because it increases HDL, the good cholesterol, but what does the alcohol do to the other cells in the body? Additionally, alcohol ingested in large amounts offsets this rise of HDL. It increases LDL cholesterol and triglycerides.

Some people may substitute smoking cigarettes or drinking caffeinated beverages for food. Both nicotine and caffeine are stimulants which cause a rise in blood glucose. The person feels energized. From where does the energy come? From body fat? No, it comes from the conversion of protein in the lean cells. Being forced to convert lean tissue cells to glucose places the liver under stress. The result is, blood cholesterol rises. Additionally, smoking creates other problems. It leads to the constriction of the blood vessels. And if the blood is high in cholesterol, the vessels can occlude and block the flow of blood.

Glen, an physician in his mid 30's, discovered his blood cholesterol was very high. He said he didn't eat breakfast, only a salad for lunch, drank coffee throughout the day and ate a large dinner at night. I suggested he eat breakfast, lunch, switch to decaffeinated coffee and add an afternoon snack. He questioned eating an egg every day and eating red meat, but agreed to eat like this for three weeks. He also began to jog on weekends. At the end of three weeks, his blood cholesterol dropped 100 points, and after six weeks it was normal.

So the question can be asked, with sugar, nicotine, caffeine and alcohol, does blood cholesterol rise because copper and other nutrients are depleted, because the pancreatic cells are sluggish or because calories are lacking?

Carbohydrates Can Reduce High Blood Cholesterol

Another nutrient people may not consume enough of, is starchy carbohydrates. People believe starches will make them gain weight. However, starchy carbohydrates must anchor each meal. The meat entree is only a decoration on the plate. All of the major health organizations suggest that carbohydrate be 55 to 60 percent of the calories. Translating those percentages into food means a woman consuming 2000 calories needs three to four servings of starch at each meal.

One benefit of starchy foods is the fiber in whole grain carbohydrates attracts and carries some of the cholesterol through the intestinal tract for excretion. The whole grains are oat bran and brown rice. The oat bran craze may have reduced blood cholesterol modestly by increasing the soluble fiber, *but it also increased the carbohydrate.* Two other benefits from the fiber in whole grains, beans, fruits and vegetables are improved bowel function and improved action of the thyroid hormone. A sluggish thyroid causes blood cholesterol to rise.

A third benefit from whole grain carbohydrates is their content of chromium, a mineral needed to lower triglycerides. A fourth benefit is that vegetables contain two nutrients, folic acid and B6, which are used by the cells to break down homocystine, an amino acid in protein foods methionine. If homocystine accumulates in the blood, blood cholesterol rises. Meats contain some vitamin B6, but cooking reduces its potency.

It might seem that one should load up with starch carbohydrates, but the cap is 55 to 60 percent of the calories. However, some books, physicians and health professionals suggest a diet with dietary fat as low as 10 percent of the calories. With protein intake kept at 15 percent, that places carbohydrate intake at 75 percent or six servings of starch foods at each meal. Aside from other problems, how comfortable would an intestinal tract be filled to bloating with fiber? Current research also shows that regardless of whether these carbohydrates are simple or complex, with this much carbohydrates, blood triglycerides will rise to unhealthy levels and HDL will drop.

Reducing Blood Cholesterol and Triglycerides

In summary, the best way to prevent high blood cholesterol and high blood triglycerides is to keep the liver healthy by eating three meals a day with sufficient calories to support lean tissue cells—spacing the meals about five hours apart.

Adults who already are experiencing high blood cholesterol, high blood triglycerides, and fatty deposits in the blood, can reduce them with the following suggestions.

Keep carbohydrates which contain adequate fiber at 55 to 60 percent and fat at 25 to 30 percent of the calories (See meal plans in Appendix).

The amount of fat at each meal should be about 22 to 28 grams of fat (depending on the total calories needed). Some can be saturated fat. However, hydrogenated and fried fats should be kept at a minimum.

Fish, preferably broiled, boiled or baked, should be eaten two to three times a week. Fish, especially deep water fish, contain Omega 3 and linolenic fatty acids which thin the blood and reduce triglycerides (See Chapter Notes for sources of linolenic acid).

Alcohol, sugar and caffeine should be consumed in moderation. The Dietary Guidelines suggest that sugar be kept to less than 15 teaspoons a day which is in one soft drink or one hard candy.

Aerobic exercise should be done three to four times a week. Aerobic exercise forces muscles to use their storage of triglycerides and stimulates LDL to be converted to HDL, (See Chapter Notes).

Medications which can produce a rise in blood cholesterol or triglycerides should be reduced or eliminated (See Chapter Notes). Often medications can be changed. A physician should be consulted. Taken together, these recommendations can improve bile function, raise HDL and lower blood cholesterol and blood triglycerides. If after four months blood cholesterol does not drop, then other causes, such as an infection or disease somewhere in the body, should be investigated.

Low Blood Cholesterol

Many people believe that the lower blood cholesterol is the better. Blood cholesterol below 120 mg/dL can indicate a medical problem. Either the liver cells are not producing enough cholesterol because the body is malnourished or the excretion rate of cholesterol is too fast, the immune system is too weak or there is an ongoing infection. People with cancer often have low blood cholesterol, are usually malnourished because they cannot eat enough food to fulfill their caloric needs to protect their immune system.

Cells without cholesterol die. One of the organs that can be short-changed is the lung. Those cells which maintain elasticity can break down, resulting in breathing difficulties and emphysema. Another organ affected is the brain. Without sufficient cholesterol, the brain cells produce less serotonin, resulting in loss of sleep, aggressive behavior and contemplation of suicide. To maintain blood cholesterol level and keep the lungs and brain healthy, the liver must be well-fed.

Cholesterol in Children

Children grow up to be adults. Isn't it a shame that 30-40 per cent of these precious people will die prematurely of heart disease? Can heart disease be prevented by mass testing or by having children consume low-fat diets? Both have been recommended by The American Heart Association (AHA) and the National Cholesterol Education Program (NCEP) (See Chapter Notes). Many adults who make decisions for children assume that if a diet is right for adults, it must be right for children. They assume that, since adults should follow a low-fat diet, so should children. They also assume that, if dietary fat and cholesterol are reduced in childhood, the risk of coronary heart disease will be reduced. However, Dr. Richard Goldbloom, professor of pediatrics at Nova Scotia's Dalhousie University of Medicine disputes this assumption.[13] He says "The validity of the assumption that putting a child, who might be at risk for coronary heart disease, on a restrictive diet all of his life to prolong it is not yet proven. People are looking for simple answers to very tough questions. They tend to believe that if they just eat "right," they will avoid heart attacks. But the issue is much more complex." To prove the assumption is right, research needs to track large numbers of children for 40 to 50 years. A study, to be completed in 1997, is to determine if dietary modifications have a detrimental effect on children's growth.

Should all children over the age of two be limited to 30 percent of their calories in fat, of which 10 percent is saturated? Why the magic age of two? It seems incongruous, on the child's second birthday, to suddenly drop the percentage of fat from 40-55 percent (the amount in breast milk and formula) to 30 percent. Such a restrictive diet beginning at this age has been questioned by the American Academy of Pediatrics' Committee on Nutrition, the major medical health group speaking on behalf of children today.[14]

Parental ignorance about the role of fat in infant nutrition seems to be widespread. A call-in survey conducted by Gerber Foods revealed that 63 percent of parents believed that what was best for them was also best for their babies. One in five parents actually restricted the amount of fat in their infant's diet.[15] T.B. Newman says in *Journal of American Medical Association*, "It is dangerous to assume that the favorable effects of reducing cholesterol in middle aged men can be generalized to children, but that the unfavorable effects cannot.[16] The implication is that children may develop harmful, unhealthy attitudes toward food. Here are some of the issues.

Ramifications of a Low-Fat Diet for Children

First, reducing dietary fat intake reduces calories. Adults are *grown*. Children are *growing* and their need for calories and nutrients are much more acute. Children require 80 to 90 calories per kilogram of weight daily, whereas adults need only 30 to 40 calories per kilogram. The additional 500 calories that a child needs daily are used to build 200,000 new cells each minute. These new cells are the foundation for organs and systems that should work for 60 years or more. From conception to the late teens, cells multiply, turn over faster, work more rapidly and are growing larger. This building program continues daily from creation to maturity-over an 18 to 20 year period.

A very important part of this building and maintenance program depends on fat and cholesterol. Cholesterol is so important for growth that during pregnancy the mother's liver increases its cholesterol production to provide, not only for herself, but for the development of her unborn baby. After birth, the child's own liver takes over. As the child grows and adds more cells, the calories and cholesterol needs increase, especially during rapid growth periods. These periods are before birth, the first two years of life, and during adolescence. Fat can provide both cholesterol and calories.

However, if a child is on a low-fat diet or too few calories, not enough cholesterol will be produced to keep up with the demand and less cells will be built. If cholesterol and calories are lacking while the brain and central nervous system are growing in number, less cells are produced. The child can become mentally impaired and the nervous system poorly developed. Other systems and organs will be retarded in growth too—heart, lungs, thyroid, adrenals, intestinal tract, etc.

Children need a higher fat diet than adults for several reasons. Fat takes up less room in the stomach, produces less carbon dioxide, and is easy on the kidney. Without fat calories, the diet must compensate with bulky carbohydrate or protein foods. With small organs and a compact body, some children are unable to consume the increased volume of food from these foods to maintain the caloric intake necessary for growth.

At four years of age, a child's stomach can only hold two cups of food or liquid. For instance, it takes an entire cup of cereal to replace the calories in two teaspoons of fat. Additionally, cereal and complex carbohydrates often make the child's stomach feel uncomfortable because the cereal contains fiber which attracts water to the gut.

Fat increases satiety. Without it, hunger sets in. What will the child eat? Sugar? This is not as bulky as cereal, but bulkier than fat. It takes three teaspoons of sugar to replace the calories in one teaspoon of fat. Additionally, sugar depletes the body of nutrients, especially zinc, necessary for growth, and copper which keep blood cholesterol levels normal. With overweight and obese children, sugar more than dietary fat will add more body fat and increase insulin resistance.

Fat is easy on small lungs. Sugar and starch produce four times more carbon dioxide than fat. That means it takes four times more calories for the small lungs to expel the carbon dioxide from carbohydrates than it does from fat. In effect, this reduces the number of calories that are available for the child's growth.

Fat is also easy on the kidneys. In place of fat calories, parents may feed their children more protein—more milk, cheese, chicken, fish, or turkey. This, however, places the kidneys under stress to excrete the waste products from the extra amino acids. Kidneys under stress can cause high blood pressure and even high blood cholesterol.

Children need dietary fat, not only from vegetable sources, but from animal sources. This is to provide the essential fatty acids and other nutrients. Any type of fat in children's diets promotes the production of bile for the liver, which we learned is necessary to carry away excess cholesterol. Additionally, foods with cholesterol happen to stimulate the production of enzymes which break down blood cholesterol and make it ready for excretion.

Many enzymes in a child's small intestinal tract are not fully developed. Therefore animal fats, like butter can be easier than vegetable fats on thier immature intestinal tract. Children placed on a low-fat, low-cholesterol diet may not receive enough calories or nutrients. Red blood cells carry oxygen. Fewer red blood cells mean less oxygen. Less oxygen translates into lower energy levels, poor attention span, and more irritability. Anemia can compromise a child's intellectual and physical potential. Parents may believe that the iron can be replaced with supplements. However, the liver, which stores iron, is small and can become overloaded quickly, causing toxicity and damage to the liver and other organs. Professional diagnosis is important before iron supplements are given. If the child has iron deficiency anemia, a safer method is for the child to eat enough food—including red meat and eggs—to support not only their lean tissue and growth, but to build and maintain red blood cells.

Less Calories, Less Energy

Some school children skip breakfast, claiming they are not hungry. This puts 18 hours between their last evening meal and lunch. If they eat very little at lunch and do not have a snack until after school, they have gone 22 hours without a good meal and without enough calories and nutrients. If a child refuses to eat in the morning, Pediatrician T. Berry Brazelton in *Touchpoint* suggests that the child may be experiencing nausea from low-blood glucose.[17] Low-blood glucose can occur if the child has not eaten for the previous 10 to 12 hours. Or the nausea may be a sign that the child had not consumed enough calories the day before to keep up with his or her activity and growth needs. The smaller liver cannot store very much glycogen, the source of glucose for the body. To correct this, Dr. Brazelton suggests serving fruit juice (without sugar) immediately upon arising, followed by breakfast 15 minutes later when blood glucose levels have stabilized and the child feels like eating. Another method is to make sure the child consumes enough food with nutrients (exclude sugar foods) for several days and note their behavior. If the child cannot eat enough to keep up with their activity output, they should cut back on their exercise time.

Sometimes children refuse to eat as a mechanism to control their environment (See Chapter Notes). This is especially true of children who are overly disciplined or feel momentarily unloved. A simple hug is a good way to reaffirm their self esteem.

A nurse told me that her two sons did not eat breakfast. She complained that they dawdled making their beds, dressing, and half heartedly ate a little breakfast. I suggested that her husband and she cuddle and hug the boys after they awoke. I also suggested some fun kind of breakfasts. It worked like a charm. When they awakened, she and her husband sat and hugged them until they squirmed away. The boys whistled, laughed and chattered away as they dressed, made their beds and ate their breakfast.

Other factors can contribute to a child's refusal to eat. Perhaps it is stress? Stress can not only be the cause of a poor appetite, but it can also increase blood cholesterol.

A divorced couple had two young daughters, each with high blood cholesterol. Since the parents had separated, the children lived with their mother during the week and with their father on weekends. Both mother and father said they provided nourishing, attractive meals, but the girls would or could not eat. A two-day food diary revealed they were eating less than 500 calories each per day. The older child's head was large for her body. The younger had lanugo hair (fine downy hair) on her arms which is often indicative of anorexia nervosa and malnourishment. Since their low-caloric intake could affect their cholesterol levels, the girls agreed to eat more, 2400 and 1800 calories respectively. The parents sought counseling. Within a few months, the girls' blood cholesterol levels dropped.

Factors that Can Lead to High Cholesterol in Children

The stress on the body from not consuming enough calories is just one factor in a child's high blood cholesterol. Look at all the factors which affect blood cholesterol in adults and consider the impact they could have on a child who is one third to one half their size. Before children are subjected to a low-fat diet or a medication, rule out the following factors.

Supplements are one factor. Because of a child's smaller body, supplements can have a greater impact and create more havoc than in an adult. For example, take vitamin C. Children only need less, 35 to 45 milligrams per day, whereas adults need 60 milligrams. Children can easily exceed the recommended dose with "enriched" canned fruits and juices and with citrus fruits or fruit juices. Instead of water, children often prefer to drink juices or juice drinks and may drink up to a quart or more a day, which can amount to over 500 mg. Because of its high acidity, the child can have a poor appetite or stomach aches. Perhaps the parent does not realize how much vitamin C their child is consuming or may not think it is a problem and insist their child take a supplement to improve their appetite. Besides, what will it do to the child's blood cholesterol, what sort of message does a child receive when they are taught to pop a pill to solve problems, nutritional or otherwise?

Mary Jane, a preschooler, was tested and her blood cholesterol was very high. Her mother and doctor were concerned. The child was scared that something awful was happening to her. She was a little "chunky," but not obese. Her mother walked with her a half hour every day. She followed an eating schedule with three low-fat meals and a snack. However, her daily intake of vitamin C was 800 mg from the enriched fruit juice. Mary Jane switched to water instead of juices, and ate more fat. Her blood cholesterol dropped to normal.

Other factors that may affect high blood cholesterol in children are medications, cigarette smoke (even secondary smoke), lack of exercise, alcohol, obesity or diabetes, anorexia nervosa, and kidney problems. Overweight children, even at 15 percent above ideal body weight, can be in the early stages of type II Diabetes and insulin resistance.

Here are some steps to help ensure that children grow and develop normally and do not develop high blood cholesterol:

- Calories and nutrients need to be adequate to support the child's lean tissue cells and their growth. Protein should be only 12 percent of calories with carbohydrates at 45-47 percent, and fat at 40 percent (See meal plans). Children can have whole milk, butter on vegetables and starches, an egg a day, and one ounce (not more) of red meat four to five times weekly until they reach the age 12 or puberty. Then they can have two ounces from the Meat Group. Fish and/or venison is recommended once or twice weekly for their omega 3 and linolenic fatty acid content.

- Exercise: Children will not only develop muscles but they will feel better about themselves if they can play physical games daily.

- Vitamin and mineral supplements are not recommended.

- Children need 9-10 hours of sleep at night because they are growing.

- Children need to drink at least 5 glasses of water daily. Milk and fruit juices can make up the other three or four.

- Sugar should be kept at a minimum and not interfere with meals or replace foods.

- Caffeine is not healthy for children. The effect on the their bodies is dose dependent, according to their size.

Children are different from adults. They are growing and have smaller organs, body mass and therefore have different needs. But like the adults, their liver never goes on vacation. If the body is fed well with enough calories and nutrients to support the work of the liver, the children will be rewarded with energy, happiness and normal blood cholesterol and triglycerides levels.

Chapter Notes:

* All questions at the beginning of this chapter are true.

1: Certain medications can increase blood cholesterol. These include amiodarone (Cordarone) a medication prescribed to counteract heart antiar-rhythmias, and glucocorticoids (Prednisone, ACTH,) given to suppress the immune functions. Drugs like estrogen and birth control pills, thiazide diuretics and beta adrenergic blockers not only raise blood cholesterol but can increase high blood triglycerides.

2: The liver produces cholesterol, a fat which is coated with protein before it enters the blood stream. The result is high density lipoprotein (HDL) and low density lipoprotein (LDL). Another fat in the blood stream is triglycerides. A cholesterol profile test records the total, HDL, LDL and triglycerides. For men upper readings are: total cholesterol 200 mg/dL, LDL 130 mg/dL and triglycerides 150 mg/dL. HDL should be higher than 35 mg/dL. The greater the HDL, the less chance of a heart attack whereas, the greater the LDL, the higher the risk. Women generally have higher levels of HDL and cholesterol, possibly because of estrogen's presence. This has been offered as a possible explanation why women, in general, until menopause have fewer heart attacks than men. Why are women subjected to the same test criteria as men? This may change now that research is underway on post menopausal women.

3: The liver receives materials from the intestinal tract, dismantles them, reforms some of them into cholesterol and triglycerides. But since these are fats, they cannot enter the watery blood stream until the liver coats them with protein making them into lipo-proteins. These lipo-proteins are carried in the blood to the cells. Muscle cells take the triglyceride part and use it for energy. All cells take the cholesterol and protein parts to build and rebuild themselves. The leftover cholesterol is picked up by the HDL and taken by the blood back to the liver where it is metabolized. Bile picks up this waste and excretes it. The excess protein and triglycerides are converted to body fat.

4: HDL Cholesterol is the good guy in the white hat. HDL keeps blood cholesterol at normal levels. It is produced in the liver and to some extent in the intestinal tract. It roams the blood stream searching for leftover cholesterol, plucking it from dying cells, from the muscle (after the triglyceride portion has been removed), and returns it to the liver where it can be reprocessed or excreted from the body. The best way to increase HDL is to exercise. Athletes have the highest HDL. Walking regularly increases HDL by 6 percent which is equal to an 18 percent drop in the risk of heart disease.

5: LDL cholesterol can be the bad guy in the black hat. When it accumulates in the blood stream, it sticks to the arterial walls, creating plaque. There are several reasons for this. The muscle may not use up the supply of LDL. The liver may fail to metabolize the returning cholesterol. The liver may fail to produce enough HDL. There may not be enough bile to collect and excrete it. Maybe there is too much fat in the diet or too little vitamin E. In any case, without an avenue of escape, the sticky LDL accumulates on the walls of the arteries, making the inside of this pipeline narrower. It is similar to what happens to old water pipes that are subjected to scaly mineral deposits from water. Water flows less easily. Blood flows less easily. Pressure builds up to pump the water or the blood through the smaller opening. (There are additional reasons for high blood pressure). Blood vessel walls become harder (atherosclerosis) making their muscles weaker. The weaker the muscles, the slower the blood flows, allowing more opportunity for LDL to stick to the walls. Additionally, the arteries of the blood stream are not like smooth glass pipes. Inside they develop scars, crevices, and bumps from the toxic oxidation of LDL where LDL cholesterol and other fats can build up, creating larger plaques.

6: Risk factors for heart disease: number one being male, next are age (55 years and over), family history of heart disease, and high blood pressure. Gender and family history are not under one's control. Many other factors are: high blood cholesterol, smoking, obesity, diabetes, lack of exercise, pregnancy, hypothyroidism, alcoholism, high stress and tension levels, chronic renal disease, obstructive liver disease, auto-immune diseases, certain medications, and electrocardiographic abnormalities.

7: The United States Department of Health and Human Services established a department called the National Cholesterol Education Program to educate people about cholesterol.

8: Both the American Heart Association and the National Cholesterol Education Program recommend several steps to reduce and prevent heart attacks. The total amount of fat no more than 25-30 percent of the calories, protein 15-20 percent, and carbohydrates 55-60 percent. Divide the fat equally between saturated, polyunsaturated, and monounsaturated. Reduce dietary cholesterol and sodium, reduce alcohol to no more than two ounces a day, exercise, stop smoking and control weight.

9: Stresses on the liver: medications, tobacco, alcohol, caffeine, vitamin C and niacin supplements, drugs, lack of food, too few calories and skipping meals, diseases of the liver, pancreas, kidney, or thyroid. An extreme example of a body not receiving enough calories and nutrients is a person with anorexia nervosa. Blood cholesterol will usually be very high. A place where people seem to feel under mental stress is at the physician's office. Their blood pressure may rise; as may blood cholesterol. This kind of high blood cholesterol is not caused by diet or a lack of exercise-it's just stress. The stress causes the blood to become more concentrated. Blood pressure and blood cholesterol (as much as 22 mg/dL) rise.

10: Copper is a necessary nutrient for many reasons. Lack of copper can cause blood cholesterol to rise, bones to demineralize, the blood to become anemic, skin and hair to lose pigmentation, brain tissue to degenerate, joints and muscles to inflame, the immune system to become vulnerable to infection, and the body to feel cold. Sources of copper are: shellfish, liver, kidney, nuts, legumes, raisins, cocoa and green leafy vegetables grown in copper-rich soil.

Copper deficiency and a drop in HDL can result from ingesting zinc supplements in amounts over the RDA (15 mg) and vitamin C in amounts over 100 mg. People take these to ward off colds because both can bolster the immune system. However, the large doses surround the cells, interfering with liver's absorption and metabolization of copper, vitamin E, medications and other nutrients. Without copper, blood cholesterol rises. Without vitamin E, LDL is oxidized, leading to plaque buildup in the blood stream.

11: Other causes of copper depletion are excessive fiber. Fiber in psyllium seeds is found in laxatives like Metamucil, and Fiberall, in bran cereals, fruits and vegetables. Copper can be depleted if a person takes calcium carbonate regularly, taken in supplement form to prevent osteoporosis and found in Caltrate, and OsCal 500. Calcium carbonate is also found in antacids such as Mylanta, Rolaids, and Extra Strength Tylenol with an antacid and Tums. More recently, Tums has been marketed to doctors and the public as a calcium supplement. But what happens to the copper?

12: To eliminate the confusion between dietary cholesterol and blood cholesterol and ensure that the public is not mislead, the United States Department of Agriculture (USDA) requires that food manufacturers refrain from using the "low cholesterol," "cholesterol free" terms without clarification and probably will ask that more emphasis be placed on the amount and kinds of fat in a product. As mentioned before, meals high in any fat can cause a rise in blood cholesterol. A teaspoon of shortening, margarine or oil is equal to a teaspoon of butter, or animal fat. Some margarines and butter (called "diet" "spread" or "whipped") have water added which reduces the amount of fat per teaspoon.

13: Sources of linol*eic* acid are: walnuts, almonds, eggs, milk (not skim milk), poultry, seeds, green leafy vegetables, vegetable oils (not olive oil). Source of linolenic acid are omega 3 oils like deep water fish like tuna, salmon, sardines, vegetables oils like soy (as long as it is not fried or hydrogenated) and canola, walnuts, wheat germ, seeds. An example of a meal plan which would supply enough linolenic is an egg for one meal, a one-half cup of 2 percent milk, whole milk or an ounce of cheese at each of three meals, two ounces of chicken, turkey or fish for one meal and a fresh green salad with 2 to 3 teaspoons of salad oil dressing at each of two meals. Substitute walnuts or almonds or seeds for salad oil.

14: Questran, Lopid, Colestid, and lovastatin such as Mevacor and Zocor. Sources of zinc: meats, fish, seafood, chicken, turkey, venison, eggs whole grains, wheat germ, fortified cereals, and oysters

15: Triglycerides are normal at 150 mg/L. Those who test out in the range of 500 to 2000 mg/L may have a genetic disposition or some disorder. Alcoholics often have blood triglycerides over 2000 mg/L. Triglyceride levels in the range of 250 to 500 mg/L can accompany obesity and diabetes. Smoking, certain medications and lack of exercise can compound the problem.

16: High triglycerides can cause acute pancreatitis and affect the beta cells that produce insulin. Symptoms of pancreatitis are severe pain in the upper abdomen and back. Pancreatitis can lead to malabsorption and diabetes mellitus.

17: Medications that increase triglycerides are: thiazide diuretics, oral contraceptives, estrogen, and beta-blocking drugs. High triglycerides can cause acute pancreatitis and affect the beta cells that produce insulin. Symptoms of pancreatitis are severe pain in the upper abdomen and back. Pancreatitis, can lead to malabsorption and diabetes mellitus. Chronic pancreatitis shows up on the an X-Ray as calcified. High blood triglycerides are present with other diseases: renal and liver diseases, and hypothyroidism

18: Omega 3 is an essential polyunsaturated fat found in fish and animals like deer that eat plants. Omega 3 tends to thin the blood and therefore can prevent clots, strokes, and heart attacks and reduce arthritic pain. It can reduce blood triglycerides in the genetically predisposed. It is recommended that all adults eat fish several times a week, a safer solution than supplements which can cause excessive thinning of the blood, blurred vision, pseudo macular degeneration and even brain hemorrhage.

19: The National Heart, Lung and Blood Institute recommends that for children the normal blood cholesterol level be 170 mg/L; above 200 mg/L is considered too high. If, on two successive measurements it is still high, then a blood cholesterol profile should be taken. Normal LDL cholesterol is 110 mg/L whereas more than 130 mg/L is considered too high. Blood tests are the only way to track blood cholesterol levels. If the child's blood cholesterol and LDL are too high, the institute recommends treatment with diet low in fat and saturated fat for one year. After six months, a second test is recommended. If the LDL cholesterol is still too high, drug therapy is recommended, but then only if the child is over ten years of age. Cholesterol-lowering drugs have serious side effects, including a lower immune system, growth deprivation, all because fat and fat soluble vitamins are not absorbed. If the cholesterol profile test reveals a high triglycerides, (over 100 mg/L) obesity may be the problem. This blood test could be used to motivate the parents and child to change their lifestyle. A very low LDL like 50 mg/L and an HDL of 20-25 mg/K should be evaluated. Such a low reading can indicate other medical problems.

20: Mass Testing of Children for Cholesterol

The American Academy of Pediatrics does not recommend mass testing for several reasons. Such testing does not always produce accurate readings, unnecessarily exciting parents and children, raising the question whether it is worthwhile to subject every child to a blood test to find the few. The Academy suggests that the child's doctor should determine the need for a blood test. It is recommended that children be tested if their grandparent or parent have a blood cholesterol in excess of 240 mg/L or have or had premature cardiovascular disease.

Secondly, how valid is mass testing? Childhood levels of blood cholesterol vary as much as 30 to 50 mg/L from day to day as their liver adjusts to the needs of the cells. Levels can ride the roller coaster before, during and after puberty.

Thirdly, unlike adults, high blood cholesterol in children does not have predictive consequences. In fact, research has shown that 80 percent of children with high cholesterol levels do not carry them into adulthood. Those that do may have been overweight or obese in childhood.

It had been reported that soldiers in the Korean war as young as 18 years of age had fatty streaks in their aortas. It was assumed if fatty streaks start in childhood they would continue into adulthood. But research has proven that these fatty streaks are intermittent and usually harmless. They may have been caused by stress. What soldier in the field is not under stress?

Whether a person is young or old, feeding the body enough calories and nutrients at each meal to support all the lean tissue cells, also, feeds the liver. The liver then will be able to provide glucose between meals, to prevent high blood cholesterol, to prevent toxins from damaging other organs, to store vitamin A, D and E, iron, copper and release them to the cells as they need them.

CHAPTER 5

Brain Power
The 100 Billion Watt Transmitter

A LTHOUGH the brain controls everything in the body, its power comes from the food the person eats. But something can go wrong with the processing of the foods and the brain will be affected.

Ask yourself what do these people have in common?

Macho males consuming 12 ounce steaks or several large cheeseburgers and a gallon of milk a day.

People trying to lose weight and drinking high-protein, low-calorie formulas or following a high-protein, low-calorie diet, or living on diet desserts and soft drinks with aspartame.

Children drinking high amounts of diet drinks and eating diet desserts and calories inadequate to support their growth.

People with many social engagements who graze at hors d'oerves buffets, eating large amounts of shrimp, cheeses, meatballs, pates, and deli meats.

What these people have in common is a stomach full of protein and a liver full of amino acids. All those amino acids in the intestinal tract are dumped on the liver and they are going to keep the liver very busy for the next few hours as it processes them. The liver will help build and rebuild cells and will convert the rest into glucose or, what is more likely, into fat. But with these many amino acids, there will be waste products which can be harmful to the kidneys and even to the brain.

The liver goes through all kinds of gyrations and uses a great amount of energy to process the amino acids. To do this, it produces hundreds, perhaps millions, of enzymes. The enzymes change the amino acids into forms which the body cells can accept.

After the amino acids are changed, the liver gathers 24 of them into protein packages which the blood delivers to the cells. These protein packages are as necessary for the cell's existence as are glucose, cholesterol, oxygen, water, vitamins and minerals (See Chapter Notes). The amount of protein picked up by the cells at any one time is very little-only what can be extracted from two to three ounces from a food in the Meat Group and a one-half serving from a food in the Milk Group.

The key here is 24 amino acids. It is all or nothing. If all 24 are not present, then the package is scrapped. The cells will not be built. The amino acids which must not be missing are one or more of the eight essential amino acids. The liver can make the other 16. But it cannot make the essential ones. Essential means they must be supplied from food and be supplied several times a day because these amino acids cannot be stored. The eight essential amino acids are found in the foods from the Meat and Milk Groups.

They can be missing if a person skips a meal or eats a meal without these foods. Cells die for the want of an essential amino acid. Some cells, especially the ones with the fastest turnover are at a greater risk than those with a slow turnover. The immune system turns over every 12 hours, the intestinal tract every two days and the bones every five or six months. Therefore the immune system is at the greatest risk for losing cells when someone skips meals or does not eat foods with some protein at each meal or eats too few calories. If calories are scarce, the body's first need is for glucose, so the protein in the meal will be converted to glucose and those amino acids are lost to the cells. Certain cells which were ready for the protein will not be rebuilt. On the flip side, when there is a surplus of protein and carbohydrate, the protein will be converted to fat.

The liver is an elegant organ which quietly goes about its work. However, such a complex system can lend itself to error. Imagine that, for some reason, the liver produces too little or none of *just one* of the many enzymes or does not have enough of the vitamins (co-enzymes) such as vitamin B6, which are needed to break down an amino acid. An amino acid is not dismantled. It is dumped back into the blood stream where it accumulates. The unclaimed amino acid circulates throughout the body, damaging cells, particularly the cells in the central nervous system and brain. If the unclaimed amino acid continues to damage the brain, the brain can become impaired and the person can develop other neurological problems, such as seizures.

Phenylalanine and the Brain

One such amino acid is phenylalanine (fennel-al-a-neen). This amino acid is necessary for growth and for appetite. The liver produces an enzyme, phenylalanine hydroxylase, which breaks down the phenylalanine, with the help of vitamin B6, into tyrosine, another amino acid. The body requires more tyrosine than phenylalanine. If there isn't enough tyrosine coming in from food, the liver will convert the phenylalanine (See Chapter Notes for functions of tyrosine).

Is the word phenylalanine unfamiliar? It can be read on the label of a product that contains aspartame (NutraSweet and Equal) "Warning . . . contains phenylalanine" (See Chapter Notes for products with aspartame). Phenylalanine and tyrosine are essential amino acids in meat, fish, poultry, eggs, milk products, dry beans and nuts.

Phenylalanine became famous in the 1950's when it was discovered that it can lead to retardation in babies who lack the enzyme. Since 1950, nearly every state tests newborns for the disorder, phenylketonuria (PKU) (See Chapter Notes). It is a rare disorder. For the one in 25,000 newborns who test positive for the PKU defect, the only recourse in preventing brain damage is to reduce the amount of dietary phenylalanine. They are started on phenylalanine-free milk and later are kept on foods low in phenylalanine (See Chapter Notes). This action has prevented countless numbers of children from being impaired.

Although it is not common public knowledge, mild cases of PKU do exist but may be asymptomatic. PKU can develop anytime in life if the liver fails to produce enough phenylalanine hydroxylase. Some precipitating events that can affect the liver's ability to produce the enzyme are: pregnancy, a medication, a disease such as rheumatoid arthritis, a connective tissue disease such as Ehlers-Danolos syndrome, or a traumatic event such as surgery, an accident, or a heart attack (See Chapter Notes). Diet too can be a factor. Malnourished people who follow low calorie diets, skip meals, or ingest aspartame can develop a mild condition of PKU.

A few years ago, a 22 year old man consulted with me. He was of medium build and wanted to lose some weight. He told me that ever since he was a little boy he took six or seven baths each day because everyone told him he smelled bad. He tried without success to date girls. I discovered that he ate little breakfast, but did eat large amounts of meat for lunch and dinner. He drank diet drinks throughout the day. I provided him with a 2200 calorie meal plan, which included very little from the meat group. I suggested he eliminate diet soft drinks. Because I believed he had several symptoms of PKU, including a short attention span, I suggested that he undergo a PKU test. Unfortunately, he did not return.

People who have a mild PKU condition are irritable, have an unpleasant body odor, are confused, forgetful, depressed, complain of headaches, memory loss, blurred vision and even have seizures (See Chapter Notes). Usually though, these signs and symptoms are not recognized as being related to diet. Instead people may have brain wave tests, an MRI, nerve tests and then a medication may be prescribed. If I were analyzing their diet, I would look for the amount of protein they are consuming, the skipped meals or adequacy of their caloric and nutrient intake and the amount of aspartame they are consuming.

Flo at 43 has been bulimic since she was about 20 years of age. When she was 14, her doctor prescribed an appetite suppressant which automatically has an effect on the central nervous system and increases heart palpitations. The medication made her confused and disoriented. She said she could not feel a needle prick in her finger when she was sewing. She also said that years later she also became confused and disoriented when she drank diet drinks or when she ate excess meat or a cup of yogurt. These reactions prompted her to switch to a vegetarian diet. She complained that she was tired all the time. When I analyzed her diet on the computer, it was too low in calories (750), too low in fat, protein and carbohydrate, sodium, potassium, iron, zinc, and the B vitamins. After she followed the meal plan that I designed for her—2000 calories with only 15 percent in protein—she reported that she had more energy, was not self destructive and could think more clearly. She also lost some excess body fat (See appendix for meal plan).

I realize I sound like I'm nagging, but when meals are skipped and the person does not consume enough calories, the protein in their lean tissue will be broken down for glucose. And when the protein breaks down it releases phenylalanine into the blood. The blood carries it back to the liver where it will need to be broken down with the aid of enzymes. However, with too few calories the liver may not have enough energy to produce the enzyme and break down the amino acid leaving it in the blood stream where it can damage the brain. Those who are at the greatest risk are children, particularly during fast growth periods when their bodies need more calories per pound. Additionally, a child's blood may accumulate too much phenylaline if they eat too much protein at a meal.

During pregnancy, more phenylalanine enters a woman's blood for her growing baby. Therefore, pregnancy is not the time to follow a low calorie diet or to skip meals, to consume too much protein or aspartame. All of these can produce an overabundance of phenylalanine. The phenylalanine accumulates in the blood, circulates to and can damage the fetus' brain. Additionally, low calorie diets precipitate the body's production of uric acid, ketones and nitrogen that also can damage the fetus's brain. A pregnant woman can prevent a lifetime of disabilities for her child if she consumes about 2200 to 2400 calories divided into three to six meals, keeps the meal servings from the meat group to 1-2 ounces and from the milk group one serving and eliminates products with aspartame and drugs. Leading obstetricians agree that pregnant women should restrict aspartame because of the changes in their bodies. However, there seems to be little concern by many doctors of pregnant women about the large amounts of phenylalanine that these women may be consuming from Meat and Milk Groups.

Some people claim they feel better when they eliminate meat and milk products, essentially living on vegetarian diets. Perhaps, they feel better because they are consuming less protein and their liver may have been deficient in the enzymes to break down certain amino acids such as phenylalanine. However, since there is no test to detect a mild form of PKU or amino acid metabolism irregularities, my assumption is conjecture. Vegetarians may feel better, but it is very difficult for them to combine foods in a meal that provides the essential amino acids and other nutrients which the

Meat and Milk Groups provide. They can receive the missing nutrients if they become lacto-ova vegetarians or fish and milk vegetarians as long as they keep the servings small and also consume, from the other food groups, the right number of calories which would keep their body from breaking down the protein in their lean tissue.

Age can make a difference in the production of enzymes. As one ages, the DNA genetic code can change, resulting in a liver gone haywire. An aging liver can produce less enzymes and what enzymes it does produce may be assigned to the wrong amino acid. Then the amino acid is not broken down and enters the blood stream to damage the brain and nerve cells. Some signs of this phenomena are, speech difficulties, loss of control of hands and limbs and memory loss (See Chapter Notes for other symptoms).

To prevent a load of protein being dumped on a poor functioning liver. I design a meal plan with less protein (10 to 12 percent of the calories) and keep the calories high enough to prevent the breakdown of protein from the lean tissue. Often making sure people have enough calories is not included when instructions are given to people such as those who have Parkinson's disease, seizures or epilepsy, brain injuries, hypoglycemia and other problems that affect the nerves and brain. I design a meal plan with less protein. To provide enough calories I increase the fat to 40 percent and keep the carbohydrates at 50 percent (See Meal Plans in Appendix). I also suggest they eliminate the aspartame. With all of this fat, can't you hear the questions about cholesterol? In my professional experience, people with the above conditions do not develop elevated blood cholesterol. My patients told me they felt and looked better, had more energy and were less stressed.

Interestingly, when I measured the patients who followed the above diet, their lean tissue increased about three to four pounds. Let me be clear about this diet. The diet does not reverse brain damage, but it did seem to improve the quality of life for my patients for the period of time I saw them. Someday soon, scientists will find a way to detect amino acid irregularities earlier in life.

College students in my nutrition class were encouraged to experiment with aspartame and large amounts of protein foods. Several students drank several quarts of milk a day. Some skipped breakfast, or ate skimpy meals. When they each followed a meal plan with about 2000 to 2600 calories daily, drank very little milk and meat and eliminated the diet drinks, some students reported changes. One woman who had endured a sinus headache for years, reported that the sinus headaches disappeared when she eliminated the aspartame. Each time she reintroduced it, they returned. Other students reported that their headaches, or mental confusion, or depression lifted when they reduced the amount of protein foods and eliminated the aspartame. Of course, not all students reported this kind of success.

Aspartame can alter the chemicals in the brain that control hunger and the desire for sweet tasting foods, particularly if taken in large quantities or without food. Since aspartame has no calories or nutrients, it is not satisfying and people eat more and gain more weight. Artificial sweeteners add body fat because their sweetness triggers the beta cells to produce the hormone insulin. The release of insulin translates into weight gain. Artificial sweeteners provide no nutrients or energy, cannot replenish liver and muscle glycogen, nor replenish the calories and nutrients needed by the liver to process the artificial sweeteners.

A woman started to gain weight and took an hour's nap every afternoon. Even though she was following the low calorie diet program, she was gaining weight. I designed a new meal plan for her. She carefully recorded what she ate and drank but she gained four pounds of fat the first week. An analysis of her beverage intake revealed what I thought was the problem, she was adding three packets of Equal to her tea, six times a day.

In place of sugar or artificial sweeteners, I suggest substituting frozen undiluted fruit juice in recipes. One tablespoon equals one third cup of sugar in sweetness. Several food companies use fruit and fruit juices to sweeten cereals, cookies, and snacks. I use it in muffins, pancakes, and breads such as banana bread (See Appendix for Recipes). Instead of soda pop or fruit drinks one can sweeten water or tea with a small amount of fruit juice.

Beware of Tyramine

Tyrosine is another amino acid the body needs. However, there may be a problem with it if foods are allowed to ferment, as when they are left on the counter to cool or they are left in the refrigerator too long. The tyrosine in the food is converted to tyramine. The tyramine must be broken down in the liver by an enzyme, monomine oxidase. There can still be a lack of the monomine oxidase. Then tyramine accumulates in the blood and one can experience bad headaches and other symptoms (See Chapter Notes for other symptoms).

If tyramine is identified as a problem, attacks can be prevented by avoiding fermented foods, glutamates like monosodium glutamate and medications which inhibit the enzyme monomine oxidase (See Chapter Notes for foods to avoid).

To ensure that people do not experience problems associated with amino acids and their breakdown, I suggest that they consume enough calories and nutrients every five hours to support their lean tissue while limiting dietary protein to 15 percent for adults and to 12 percent for children at each meal. Then the liver will be well fed and healthy and can keep up with the demand for the enzymes. Care should also be taken with fermented and leftover foods as suggested in Chapter 12.

The Desire to Be Healthy

Ask yourself what these people have in common:

Macho males eating large dishes of spaghetti with meat sauce, people eating foods with enough calories and nutrients and exercising to lose weight, children drinking diluted fruit juice and eating fruit for dessert, and people at social engagements grazing from a buffet of fruits, vegetables and sandwiches.

What they have in common is keeping their livers well fed, preventing the liver from being overloaded with amino acids and Eating for the Health of It.

Chapter Notes:

1: All 24 amino acids, including the eight essential ones, are present in animal foods. These are known as complete proteins. Plant foods are incomplete proteins because they contain fewer essential amino acids.

2: Tyrosine is necessary for many actions in the body. It helps the brain transmit messages, helps the thyroid regulate metabolism, helps the adrenal glands regulate breathing and heart rate and helps produce pigment for the eyes and skin to protect them from the sun's rays.

3: Aspartame is an additive in about 96 percent of all diet soda pop. Government guidelines say aspartame must be listed even if a tiny amount is added. Aspartame replaces sugar in cocoa mixes, vitamin supplements, chewing gum laxatives, and in low calorie or sugar free desserts such as frozen yogurt, ice cream, puddings, gelatin, and many other uncooked products. Phenylalanine and another amino acid, aspartic acid, are used with alcohol and methanol to make aspartame. It is sold as "NutraSweet" and "Equal" and is 150 to 200 times sweeter than sugar. The liver needs to produce alcohol dehydrogenase to break down methanol glycol in aspartame and this action requires copper. Amino acids such as aspartame, are treated by the Food and Drug administration as foods. Thus, companies manufacturing products containing these chemicals are not required to list a warning of possible adverse reactions, hypersensitivity or contraindication. An exception is made for aspartame. It must print a warning "Phenylketonurics: contains phenylalanine."

4: To prevent mental retardation and death, every state has a program for testing newborn babies in the United States a few days after drinking milk. The blood test detects the large amounts of phenylalalanine. It is not sensitive to small amounts. The amount over 15 to 20 mg/dL identifies the genetic disease, phenylketonuria (PKU). One in every 12,000 to 25,000 newborns in the U.S. is affected annually. Some babies are not tested, especially if they go home from the hospital one or two days after birth. At least two states, Vermont and Maryland, have a voluntary testing program and some states have a provision which allows parents to decline testing of their newborns on religious grounds. Another amino acid, tyrosine, is also lacking in those with PKU so the babies are fed a formula with tyrosine added and phenylalanine stripped from the milk protein. Research indicates that those diagnosed with PKU must continue this special diet indefinitely. However, as PKU children approach their teen years, many revolt against their childhood diet. With the increase in phyenylalanine consumption, they become more destructive and more mentally impaired.

5: Other symptoms of an accumulation of phenylalanine in the blood are speech difficulties, loss of control of hands and limbs, depth perception, and memory, hypoglycemia, an allergic reaction, the flu like symptoms, or medications. Medications can interfere with enzyme production. Some drugs to control high blood pressure act on the brain. This may cause an increased reaction to aspartame and high protein diets.

6: Symptoms of excess tyramine: the blood vessels can constrict and a person can develop a migraine headache, high or low blood pressure, nausea, heart palpitations, vomiting, numbness, dizziness, and tingling in the fingers and toes.

7: Preventing the build up of tyramine in foods.

Tyramine content in a food can increase when protein or beverages ferment over time in a warm room. Cooking of the fermented food will not destroy the tyramine content.

To Prevent the Fermentation of Foods:

- Refrigerate perishable items immediately after purchase and consume within 48 hours.
- Refrigerate foods immediately after serving and consume within 48 hours.
- Use only clean utensils and clean hands when dishing up the food.

- Use care when eating out: Choose plain and simple dishes rather then casseroles or dishes with sauces. Choose vinegar and oil rather than mixed salad dressings, which can contain monosodium glutamate.

Foods to Avoid:

- Fermented cheeses
- Wines, beer, alcohol, ale, apple cider
- Smoked or pickled fish, caviar, anchovies
- Chopped liver, and pates, dry or semi-dry sausages (pepperoni) tenderizers, marinated meat, meat extracts
- Yeast cake
- Soy sauce
- Worcestershire sauce
- Sauerkraut, tomato juice, ripe avocado
- Fermented fruits, ripe bananas, pineapple and raisins
- Fresh raspberries, canned figs, sour cream, buttermilk, yogurt, peanuts chocolate, coffee, tea, caffeine beverages sour dough bread.

8: Additives and drugs that can elicit the same symptoms as a build up of tyramine: Monosodium glutamate (MSG), a synthetic amino acid is a flavor enhancer. It stimulates the taste buds and can affect brain and nerve cells. Some of the symptoms that characterize a MSG symptom are: headache, numbness in the back of the neck, radiating to the arms and back, burning sensation in back of neck. forearms, and chest, chest pain, tightness and flushing of the face and upper body, dizziness, drowsiness, rapid heart beat, weakness and nausea which occurs from 1 to 6 hours after eating. MSG is added to Chinese foods, foods at fast food restaurants and to many processed foods: chips, soups, salad dressings, sauces, frozen meals, diet foods, lunch meats, peanuts, poultry injected with broth. You can buy items for your home that contain MSG: Accent, Zest, Subu or seasoning salts. Read the label. Always ask at a restaurant if the chef adds MSG to the foods or which foods do not have it. If you will have a meal aboard an airline, call ahead and ask them to serve your food without MSG. If monosodium glutamate is added to a product, in the past it was also known as: "hydrolyzed vegetable or plant protein," "natural flavors" or "natural flavoring." But now, the regulations by the FDA say it must be listed as monosodium glutamate.

CHAPTER 6

Too Much Fuel Or Not Enough
The Blood Sugar (Glucose) Story

DIABETES. What does it bring to mind? Someone who loses weight too fast, is very thirsty or injects insulin? This describes one type of diabetes (Type I) which develops suddenly and afflicts one million people in this country. But another type of diabetes, Type II, afflicts 20 times more people. And the numbers are growing, keeping pace with the numbers of people who have become overweight and obese. Being overweight is the greatest risk factor for Type II Diabetes, especially for the obese and overweight women who make up 60 percent of this category. Type II Diabetes is more insidious, harder to detect, and harder to control than many other diseases.

In the United States, Type II Diabetes is the fourth direct cause of death but, because it leads to many other diseases, it indirectly translates to a much higher death rate.

Diabetes, whether it is Type I or Type II is a condition in which glucose molecules accumulate in the blood because many cells cannot absorb them. In Type I Diabetes, the result of a genetic disorder, lean and fat cells are lost quickly. But Type II Diabetes is usually the result of an environmental impact. Lean cells are lost but fat cells are gained. Since Type II Diabetes is hard to control, prevention is the key.

Blood Glucose: Fuel for the Body

Most of us enjoy well controlled blood glucose levels and never think about it. Whether we are asleep or awake, walking or running, sitting or eating, glucose steadily (24 hours a day) moves into the cells to maintain the level of fuel. And blood carries it there. The sources of blood glucose are food, glycogen stored in the liver and protein from lean tissue cells. The number of glucose molecules that the blood carries at any one time is determined by several mechanisms: the interaction of three hormones, what we eat and drink, how much and when, and what kind of exercise, how often and for how long.

Fuel Control

Insulin is the most predominate of the three hormones, But the other two, adrenaline and glucagon, are also important. They keep insulin in line (See Chapter Notes). Glucose is digested from certain foods in the intestinal tract and then enters the blood stream. As blood glucose rises above 90 to 110 mg/dL, insulin comes into play. Insulin is "programmed" to reduce the number of glucose molecules in the blood in three steps. It carries glucose into the cells for use as energy or to the cells in the liver and muscles where it is stored as glycogen, and excess glucose is converted to body fat (triglycerides). While there is a limit on the amount of glycogen that can be stored in the cells, there is no limit on the amount of fat the cells can store (See Chapter Notes).

For insulin to carry glucose into the cells, certain vitamins and minerals must be present. One vitamin needed is vitamin B6 which is provided by vegetables. Three minerals needed are copper, zinc, and chromium which are provided by from the meat, whole grains and vegetables (See Chapter Notes).

Insulin would continue taking glucose out of the blood if it weren't for the other two hormones, glucagon (also made in the pancreas) and adrenaline (made in the adrenals). They are activated when the number of glucose molecules drops below 90 mg/dL which occurs from about two hours to two and one half hours after a meal. Glucagon and adrenaline trigger the liver cells to release *more* glucose into the blood. These particular glucose molecules do not come from food. They come from either the liver's storage of glycogen (its backup source of fuel) or from the liver's conversion of the protein from lean tissue cells. Glucose to replenish blood glucose cannot come from the glycogen stored in the muscles. The glycogen stored in the muscles protects vitial organs such as the heart and lungs. However, the protein in the muscles *can* be tapped to replenish blood glucose. Muscles are a large source. Muscles make up 45 percent of the lean tissue in the body. But when they lose protein, they become weaker.

If something goes wrong with one of the hormones blood glucose is affected. In Type I Diabetes, the beta cells that produce insulin have either been damaged or destroyed, so there is little or no insulin to carry glucose into the cells. In Type II Diabetes, the beta cells are producing insulin, but the cells are not accepting it or the production of insulin is sluggish. In both Type I and II, glucose accumulates in the blood.

Type II Diabetes is difficult to detect in the early stages with a fasting blood glucose (See Chapter Notes). A full blown case may take years to develop. However, there are some warning signs.

One sign is fast weight gain (especially if the weight settles around the abdomen). Men who allow their waists to grow to 40 to 68 inches are five to seven times more likely to develop diabetes than those with waists measuring 27-34 inches. In men, the cause of excess weight is often beer and alcohol, whereas, in women the cause is often alcohol, overeating, and inactivity. In my experience and from reports in the medical literature, adults seem to increase body fat faster after their percent of body fat reaches 20 percent. People reported to me that they gained weight, even though they did not change their food habits and ate less calories. Such a case was George who was surprised to learn he had diabetes.

George, a patient of mine, developed Type II Diabetes. He noticed after reaching 40 years of age that it was easier to add weight. When he was 44, he realized he hadn't been feeling well and wasn't his usual affable self with the retarded children he taught. His physician discovered that George's blood glucose was 240 mg/dL two hours after eating. He prescribed hypoglycemic medication and told George to lose weight.

George had no warning of his impending diabetes—no excessive thirst, urination or weight loss as do those who depend on insulin injections. He didn't develop the ketoacidosis that Type I patients do. His pancreas was producing insulin. Yet, he was encountering the same problems as does someone without insulin. Glucose was rising (hyperglycemia) in the blood and so was the insulin.

Other signs of Type II Diabetes are generalized itching, numbness in the fingers and toes, yeast infections and muscle weakness. As Type II Diabetes progresses, adults may develop a characteristic shape with fat gained around their middle, a loss of muscles, especially evident in their flat buttocks, thin legs and small thighs—all are signs of lean tissue loss.

The extra body fat seems to trigger the body to build a rigid wall around cells in the liver and muscles. When insulin arrives at the cell door with glucose and protein to store glycogen, it cannot enter. So glucose molecules collect in the blood. Faced with a rising number of glucose molecules, insulin's only choice is to convert the extra molecules to triglycerides or body fat creating a vicious cycle for those with Type II Diabetes. More weight is gained.

The Increase in Type II Diabetes

Type II Diabetes is a growing concern in the United States. In the past 40 to 50 years the number of adults and children who have developed it, has ballooned to 20 times more cases than Type I. The number has kept pace with the increasing numbers of over-weight people (See Chapter Notes). In fact, in 1980, 25 percent of the population was overweight, whereas, today it is 33 percent.

Type II Diabetes doesn't just begin in adulthood. It can begin at any age. In fact, the next generation's risk of developing Type II Diabetes is of great concern. Newborns who weigh more than nine pounds are at great risk. Even when born with few fat cells and low birth weight, they can gain fat cells if their parents force them to finish the bottle or start them on solid food too early. Fat cells are laid down in great numbers during the first year of life.

In fact, infants at one year of age are 50 percent heavier today than those of a generation ago. Is this because babies are started on solid foods and formulas when they are only a few weeks to a few months old? Can this be at least one reason why, in the United States today, 10 to 12 percent of all school age children are over-weight? Whereas 40 to 50 years ago an obese child was a rarity.

Why is the increase in Type II Diabetes such a new phenomena? Is it lack of physical exercise? Generations ago, very few people were overweight. If they were, it was a sign of affluence or their station in life. It meant they did not have to do physical work to survive. People walked everywhere. Today, Americans drive or are driven to work or school, to the mall, to the restaurants, the supermarkets, church, to a gym to exercise on machines. They ride lawnmowers, use the remote for TV and sit watching others compete in games. They sit and sit and sit. Advertisers clamor for their fast food dollars, dollars which buy foods high in fat, sugar, or sodium. Many children are idle too, dining on cartoons and fast foods, sugary foods, salty snacks and playing games that exercise the fingers and not the feet. Most are either bussed or driven to school. "It is well known that mass obesity in our society is primarily caused by physical inactivity rather than excess calories," says Researcher Dr. Arthur Leon.[18]

Inactivity means less oxygen intake. Yet oxygen is necessary to ignite glucose from food, burn up body fat and create energy, just as oxygen is needed to ignite gasoline and make a car move. Part of the problem is the reduced amount of oxygen in the environment. Before the industrial revolution, the air was not very polluted. Today, the air is more polluted both indoors and out. One of these pollutants is cigarette smoke. Oxygen intake is further restricted if a person is under stress, has asthma, a blockage of the respiratory tract, or extra body fat that squeezes up against the diaphragm.

It Doesn't Always Take Calories to Gain Weight

Without much oxygen to ignite glucose, the person with Type II Diabetes does not have much energy. Nor does the liver store much glycogen which normally supplies glucose between meals. About two hours after they have consumed a meal, their blood glucose drops. The person with Type II Diabetes feels weak and hungry and wants to grab anything for a quick boost. Many patients have told me they have a overwhelming craving for sweets. They may choose products which contain calories or, what is more likely today, products which contain artificial sweeteners.

Some people believe that artificial sweeteners are harmless and do not add body fat because they contain no sugar or calories. Certainly, advertisements play on this theme. Artificial sweeteners, because of their sweet taste, turn on the insulin hormone which for someone with Diabetes Type II can add more body fat. Body fat is very ineffective as a source of glucose between meals since only a tiny fraction, five to seven percent, can be converted. Blood glucose drops. Since artificially sweetened products do not physically satisfy, people tend to eat more. The more frequently they consume artificial sweeteners, the more opportunity insulin has to add body fat. What all this means is that artificial sweeteners can help make a person fat despite all the popular notions to the contrary.

It isn't necessarily calories that make people gain weight. It is how the hormones which control blood glucose are affected. Similar hormonal reactions occur when people ingest caffeine or medications, none of which contain calories. Caffeine stimulates the adrenals to release glucose. The beta cells respond and release insulin. It isn't the occasional ingestion of caffeine that causes the problems with the hormones. It is the yo yo ingestion all day, every day that yank the hormones around. After several years of being overstimulated, beta cells can "wear out," become sluggish or exhausted. Then a person may develop Type I Diabetes—dependent on insulin injections.

Medications to control Type II Diabetes also affect the hormones. A class of hypoglycemic medications reduce blood glucose (See Chapter Notes) but they may increase the problem. They stimulate the beta cells to produce more insulin, forcing the glucose out of the blood by converting it to fat. Glycogen is not stored. Body fat is. Diabetes grows worse with additional body fat. After five to ten years of being overstimulated by the hypoglycemic medications the beta cells can become exhausted, forcing reliance on insulin injections. But again, injecting insulin also may produce more body fat and more hypoglycemic symptoms. Since some researchers have reported more deaths from heart disease with hypoglycemic medications than with diet alone, hypoglycemic medications may not be the answer for everyone. In my opinion, a better solution is a drug for overweight people or those with Type II Diabetes, which stimulates the liver and muscle glycogen storing cells to pick up the extra blood glucose so it can used for energy between meals and is not converted to body fat. A new drug, glucophage, is designed to do just that, but should be used cautiously.

Other medications can lead to weight gain and if a person has a genetic predisposition, the weight gain may lead eventually to Type II Diabetes (See Chapter Notes for the list of medications that can cause weight gain).

One of these medications is a class of diuretics used to reduce water accumulation and high blood pressure. People who restrict their calories not only lose lean tissue cells but also lose potassium. Potassium balances with sodium. When potassium is lost sodium is left holding the bag of water outside the cell. Water gathers in the fingers, ankles and elsewhere blood pressure rises. Blood thickens. Nerve and brain cells may be affected.

In an overweight person, diuretic and beta blockers (another blood pressure medication) may cause them to gain body fat. A vicious cycle ensues. Fortunately, there are blood pressure medications which do not cause a gain in body fat (See Chapter Notes).

Sugar and alcohol also stimulate the beta cells to release insulin.

The Difficulty With Losing Weight

With the accumulation of body fat, many overweight people try to lose weight. They may choose products low in fat and calories, take appetite suppressants, buy into weight loss programs, consume fewer calories, go without meals, and they may even exercise. In the United States, people are spending about $33 billion a year on devices, fitness clubs, and low calorie foods. But often if they lose weight, especially people with Type II Diabetes, the weight returns within a year.

A consequence of skipping meals and following a low calorie diet is the stress it produces in the body. Stress triggers the adrenal hormone to raise blood glucose, just as it does with caffeine, alcohol, and some medications. With the rise of blood glucose, insulin is released and shortly after, a sudden drop in glucose occurs (hypoglycemia). The person can experience an unexplained anxiety attack which can come "right out of the blue" scaring the "living daylights" out of them. Or they may experience a major headache or depression (Other symptoms are listed in the Chapter Notes). These symptoms can be so disabling that a person may seek help from a psychologist, psychiatrist or their family physician. Usually they are told that they have a chemical imbalance. A medication, such as a tranquilizer or an anti-depressant, is prescribed, many of which affect the hormones that control blood glucose. The person feels better but he or she may start to gain weight. The real solution is for people with Type II Diabetes to change their lifestyle.

The DEET Program

A program which people with Type II Diabetes or people who are gaining water weight or are having anxiety attacks can follow is called the DEET program. But the longer a person waits to begin the program, the more difficult it becomes. Persistence, patience, and motivation are required because it may take several months to several years to make the new regime a way of life. The goals are to avoid alerting or awakening the beta cells to produce insulin, and to use up as much glucose and fatty acids in the blood as possible before they turn to fat. The result is a loss of body fat (not lean tissue weight). Does it require a change in lifestyle? Probably! Is it worth it? Assuredly yes! Controlling body fat weight can prevent many other diseases including heart disease and strokes which increases medical costs and reduces the quality of life.

DEET means: **D**iet, **E**liminate the offending substances, **E**xercise, and **T**esting the blood. The DEET program is like a four legged stool. Take one leg away and the program collapses.

Diet: Eat six small meals every two and one half hours to prevent the breakdown of lean tissue cells (See Appendix for meal plan).
Eliminate: Eliminate substances that overstimulate the beta cells (See Chapter Notes).
Exercise: Exercise after each meal for 10 to 15 minutes, more if possible. Aerobic exercise uses glucose and the free fatty acids in the blood for energy. Exercise also makes the muscles and liver cells accept glucose. The result is less glucose in the blood and more stored in the liver and muscle cells.
Test: Test the blood for the level of glucose at regular appropriate intervals.

DIET

The meals are divided into six meals a day. Each small meal is 350 to 400 calories, consumed every two and one half hours to three hours and is comprised of foods chosen from all six food groups. The goal is to prevent hunger and cravings for offending substances and to provide the body with all 60 nutrients and enough calories to prevent the loss of lean tissue (See sample meals in Appendix).

ELIMINATE

The substances to eliminate are those which raise blood glucose precipitously and alert or stimulate the beta cells to produce insulin (See Chapter Notes).

EXERCISE

In Type II Diabetics and overweight people who have difficulty losing weight, the cells resist insulin. They accept insulin when exercise is regular (five times a week), of low intensity, and long (an hour at a time). Endurance exercise with deep breathing can increase the capacity of the lungs and force more oxygen into the body cells. Oxygen and glucose burn up body fat. Regular aerobic exercise can also decrease blood triglycerides and LDL cholesterol and increase HDL cholesterol.

In my experience with people who have type II Diabetes, the best results for weight loss seem to occur when people exercise 40 minutes per 130 pounds daily. The trick in type II Diabetes is to time the exercise when glucose is rising and the cells are resisting insulin. Glucose rises immediately after a meal or a snack. Therefore, it is more logical to exercise after the meal. Using my formula, a 350 pound person would need to exercise one and one-half hours daily, or 30 minutes after each meal. Because of the heavy body weight, exercise should be slow, steady, easy, and one that a person can enjoy and do the rest of his or her life. With this method, my Type II Diabetes patients shed fat faster and kept it off more successfully than those who exercised only 30 minutes once a day. The people who exercised more lost as much as three pounds of fat weekly, even though they were eating 2000 or more calories a day. They also avoided the drawn look and hanging flesh so characteristic of a person who follows a low calorie diet. Dr. M.N. Kaplan, in the *American Journal of Cardiology,*[19] says that it may be true that for cardiovascular fitness a person may only need 30 minutes of exercise a day. But for weight loss and loss of abdominal fat, a person needs an hour.

When people exercise they should drink a glass of water every fifteen minutes. I also suggest plenty of water during the day (See Chapter eleven).

TEST

Testing blood glucose daily, maybe even several times daily, can give people with Type II Diabetes an idea of the impact various substances, exercise, and meals have on their blood glucose. Testing does not need to be continued each day but should be conducted at least once a week.

Many of my Type II Diabetic patients, like George below, have followed this DEET program religiously. They claim they were not tempted by sweets, nor were they hungry between meals. They said they felt healthier. They lost weight and their blood tests improved. Because of their success, they were more motivated to stay with the meal and exercise program (See meal plan in Appendix).

George, over 40 and overweight, is an example of someone who controlled his Type II Diabetes. I provided him with an exercise regime and enough calories—2000—to protect his lean tissue cells. I encouraged him to eliminate those substances that cause a precipitous rise in blood glucose. He started on this regime in the fall. It was right on the heels of when he had built a large beer barrel in his bar near the television set where he gathered on Saturdays with his buddies. He found it almost impossible to give up beer but disciplined himself to do so. At Christmas, the focus switched to wine. On New Year's Eve, it was champagne. With encouragement, he took control of the alcohol situation, adhered to the diet and walked an hour each evening after dinner. By Easter, he had lost 40 pounds of fat, was off the anti-diabetic medication and looked healthy. Two years later, during a chance encounter, he smiled broadly. He was happy, laughed about the alcohol and said if it hadn't been for my nagging, he would probably still have diabetes.

It wasn't just the alcohol restriction that controlled George's diabetes without the medication. It was George's determination, the encouragement he saw from the loss of body fat which we measured each time he came for an appointment and the support he received from his family, his physician, and his dietitian. It was also his understanding of the importance of combining foods on a timely basis, of testing his blood glucose, and of exercising after meals. He also had the type of diabetes in which most of the pancreatic cells are still producing insulin. He also did not delay losing body fat when Type II Diabetes was first diagnosed.

In conclusion, it is difficult to control Type II Diabetes even if you do completely change your lifestyle. Prevention is certainly easier. The most important factors in maintaining ideal body weight is including daily aerobic exercise and eating just the right number of calories to support lean tissue. Those who gain ten excess pounds of fat (except pregnant women) can lose them by following the DEET program without needing to test their blood.

Gestational Diabetes

There is another type of diabetes which is similar to Type II Diabetes. It develops during pregnancy and is called Gestational Diabetes. The outward sign for the woman is a gain of several pounds in one week. Normally, a pregnant woman should gain a steady three quarters of a pound per week. Women who are at the greatest risk for gestational diabetes are those who are overweight or obese, have had difficulty losing weight after a previous pregnancy or are older. Delivering a baby over nine pounds and developing Gestational Diabetes can be a warning that the woman may develop Type II Diabetes five to ten years later. The nine pound newborn is also at risk later in his or her life.

Gestational Diabetes is a serious condition for the woman and her baby. The fetus is at risk for mental impairment and deformities. To prevent these disabilities in the future, Dr. Roger Mazze of the Mayo Clinic in Rochester, Minnesota,[20] believes that all women with Gestational Diabetes or women who deliver a baby over nine pounds be examined yearly and given a two or three hour glucose tolerance test to detect the early stages of Type II Diabetes. If the woman has Type II Diabetes, she can take action to prevent placing her next baby at risk.

Preventing Disabilities

When a woman notices she has gained several pounds of weight in one week, she should see her physician immediately to prevent her baby from being born with disabilities. Her body began to change as soon as she became pregnant. More estrogen is being produced. More glucose is being produced. The beta cells are under the gun to produce more insulin to take the glucose into the newly forming cells. The woman's gain in weight is a sign that her beta cells are too sluggish and not producing enough insulin to match the increased amount of glucose entering the blood. Without enough insulin, glucose accumulates in the mother's blood and is converted to fat instead of entering the fetus' cells. The fetus does not grow or develop normally.

To prevent damage to the fetus, the woman with Gestational Diabetes is started on a program similar to the one for Type II Diabetes, except for three differences. She needs to test her blood and urine several times a day. She needs to give herself insulin injections (See Chapter Notes). And she needs to increase her caloric intake 300 calories, distributed over six meals.

Exercise during pregnancy is very important. It benefits not only her baby but herself. The cells can accept the insulin better and therefore the glucose enters the fetus' cells and is not converted to her body fat. It also strengthens the muscles used in delivery. A woman's progress during pregnancy is usually evaluated by weight alone. But a more exact evaluation is to distinguish how much of the weight gain is body fat and how much is lean tissue.

Just because a woman is overweight or believes she is, pregnancy is not the time to diet. Dieting is for the time when she is not starting the life of another. During pregnancy, the fetus competes with the mother for glucose and protein. If the mother restricts her food intake, the mother's lean tissue and body fat create toxins, uric acid, ketones and fatty acids. These by-products enter the blood and damage the fetus' brain. Even if she is not dieting, the risk of these by-products entering her blood stream during pregnancy are possible. She will need to keep an eye out for them by testing her urine and blood several times a day. If ketones are present or blood glucose registers over 150 mg/dL, she can check three things. Is she consuming enough calories from the six food groups at each meal? Is she injecting enough insulin? Is she exercising after meals?

Women want to have healthy babies, but they may not know the dangers of being overweight or using pregnancy to lose weight. When they are counseled on the DIEET program, and follow it for the nine months out of their lifetime, they can prevent a lifetime of disabilities for their child and a lifetime of heartaches.

Diabetes Type I

TYPE I Diabetes is very different from Type II Diabetes. Type I is almost like a different disease. In Type I, the symptoms usually develop suddenly and usually in childhood or the early twenties. In Type I Diabetes, the beta cells which produce insulin have been destroyed for some reason (See Chapter Notes for the causes of Type I Diabetes) and weight, both body fat and lean, is lost at a fast rate. Consulting a physician is critical (See Chapter Notes).

However, Type I can also come on slowly at any time in life. So don't be too misled by the commonly acknowledged signs of Type I. The symptoms are so similar to those accompanying other diseases that it is difficult to recognize Type I Diabetes. The signs and symptoms are nausea, vomiting, lethargy, urinary tract infections, vaginal infections, etc. (See Chapter Notes for other symptoms). If several of these signs and symptoms are present, a physician should be consulted.

In Type I as in Type II Diabetes, the liver and muscles cannot take up their share of glucose without insulin. Therefore, the number of glucose molecules rises in the blood. The liver and muscle cells are starving and signal the liver to send more glucose. This just makes things worse. The liver converts the protein from lean tissue to glucose. Because insulin is not carrying glucose or protein into the liver and muscle cells, the cells are not rebuilt. Muscles become wasted and lean tissue is lost. With the breakdown of lean tissue and fat, undesirable products (uric acid, ketones, fatty acids, and potassium) pollute the blood stream. It is like dirty water going through the pipes to a human filtering plant (the kidneys).

Water is extracted from the cells in an attempt by the body to dilute and rid the blood of this dirty material. The person is very thirsty, urinates excessively, loses weight (lean tissue cells), and becomes dehydrated. When cells are lost, so is potassium, leaving, sodium holding the bag of water outside the cell wall. Feet swell. Vision is distorted and blurry. The breath smells fruity. Blood thickens. Blood pressure rises. All this accumulation of acid in the blood is caused by the loss of the balancing alkaline substances and it leads to ketoacidosis, consulting a physician is critical.

Carlene, A high school senior, developed diabetes dramatically. She told me that for years she skipped meals, ate few calories all day to remain thin. Suddenly, one day her vision became blurry, she was very thirsty, urinated excessively and began to lose weight quickly. Her fasting blood glucose tested over 400 mg/dL. Her doctor diagnosed Type I diabetes. Usually, patients with Type I Diabetes are hospitalized to regulate and adjust the amount of insulin dosages to control blood glucose. But Carlene refused. She believed that she could regulate her blood glucose within the normal range by diet and exercise alone-no insulin. Her doctor and I were skeptical. However, Carlene followed the 2000 calorie diabetic meal plan and the exercise regime that I designed for her. Almost immediately, her blood glucose level normalized. Her mood improved, a change observed by her family and boyfriend. She was able to control her blood glucose without insulin, at least for the few months that I followed her case. However, the prognosis for controlling Type I Diabetes solely with diet and exercise is highly risky to say the least; I suspected she may have been experiencing what physicians call the "honeymoon period." Her physician said she would eventually need insulin injections.

Health is always at risk when lean tissue cells are lost. With diabetes, people cannot take chances. When diabetes is uncontrolled, their blood cholesterol and triglycerides rise and plaques can accumulate in the arteries, a forerunner to heart disease. Additionally, they have poor circulation, a forerunner to impotence and blindness. Poor circulation can also result in the amputation of a leg. Pregnant women can develop ketones in their blood and damage their unborn babies. The immune system can weaken, resulting in more frequent illnesses and infections. If blood glucose remains high, the sweet environment of the body fluids can allow yeast to grow and cause vaginal and urinary tract yeast infections.

But none of these health problems need develop if people with Type I Diabetes learn about the disease, are persistent, follow the DIEET program and have an optimistic view of life (See Chapter Notes on the DIEET Program). They can learn to control their diabetes before it controls them.

Carlene was motivated to bring her diabetes under control from the beginning. But the question for her and for anyone with diabetes is, can they continue to be motivated and to discipline themselves to test their blood glucose, follow a fairly strict regimen of diet, insulin injections, and exercise daily for the next 50 years? Carlene can never again skip meals or follow a low calorie diet as she once did if she wants to live a good quality life and have as much fun in life as someone who does not have diabetes. She can be healthier than people who have not developed as healthy a discipline toward food and exercise as she has been forced to do.

Jan age 28, has Type I Diabetes. On her own she tried to control her blood glucose with only fair success. She had had diabetes since childhood. She said that while she was growing up, her doctor couldn't provide answers and neither she nor her parents knew where to go for help. By trial and error, she developed her own regime of glucose control. She chose the kind of exercise she enjoyed and chose what to eat and when. She kept detailed records. While she believed others blamed her for her lack of control over the diabetes, she later discovered she lacked correct information.

After marrying and giving birth to a child, she enrolled in my nutrition class as part of her nurse's training program. There she discovered she was correctly eliminating sugar, alcohol and cigarettes. She also was exercising—swimming everyday. But she did not feel well and could not control the rise of glucose molecules in her blood. An analysis of her diet revealed she was eating meals on time, but her diet consisted of too much protein, too little carbohydrate, diet soft drinks with caffeine and only 1200 calories daily. I suggested she increase the calories, the complex carbohydrates, and eliminate the caffeine.

I next saw her three years later. She had lost a great deal of weight and was down to only 12 per cent body fat. Her new doctor had prescribed extra vitamins and minerals and restricted her caloric intake to 1200 a day, a regime that she was following religiously. When she developed edema and high blood pressure, he prescribed medications. Still, her blood glucose levels were erratic and she didn't feel well. She reported that she experienced flatulence, bloating and cramps. I measured her for body fat and lean tissue weight and then designed a 2200 calorie diet for her. I suggested she drink lactose reduced milk and eliminate the aspartame. She began to feel better. Her blood glucose normalized. The edema left her hands and feet, her abdomen became flat. After a few weeks, she was able to discontinue the medications (not the insulin). She gained five pounds of lean tissue weight and only two pounds of body fat. She discovered independently that the high potency vitamins increased her blood glucose level; I thought they also may have irritated her intestinal tract. Today she has more control over her diabetes, seldom needs to call the doctor for insulin adjustments, and is not a passive participant in her health. And she has stayed thin and healthy.

Jan lives a fairly normal life, as can anyone with the insulin-dependent type of diabetes. She swims every day for 30 to 40 minutes, and eats a meal every five hours. She has learned she can consume 2000 calories a day and still stay thin. By consuming enough starch carbohydrates and calories, more glycogen can be stored in the liver. A liver full of glycogen from complex carbohydrates can maintain a steady blood glucose level while requiring less insulin (See Chapter Notes).

The DIEET Program

Jan uses a four-legged stool technique: Diet, Insulin injection, Exercise, and Testing (DIET). I prefer to add another "E" for "Eliminating the counter productive substances." The DIEET program is similar to the Type II Diabetes program except those with Type I must give themselves injections of insulin.

Diet

To keep the liver pantry filled with glycogen, most women need at least 2000 calories, others may need as many as 2400 calories depending on the weight of their lean tissue. Men need between 2200 to 2800 calories. These calories are divided into three meals to be consumed no more than five hours apart. The calories are parceled out for each meal into 15 percent protein, 25-30 percent fat, and 55-60 percent carbohydrates, a recommendation from the American Diabetes Association (See meal plans in appendix).

However, some people, especially teenagers and young women, are afraid to eat a lot of food. They may even use their diabetes to lose weight by discontinuing the insulin injections. This, of course, is a highly dangerous practice. They can quickly slip into ketoacidosis and require hospitalization. Some diabetics may continue to put their bodies through these episodes because the need to control other people or the need for attention or the fear of becoming fat is stronger than the fear of dying or threat of losing a kidney or eyesight. They also may be rebelling against a disease which dominates their lives. To help them accept the disease and care for themselves, they may need the help of not only a registered dietitian but a psychiatrist or psychologist.

Several researchers have suggested that eating disorders be considered in women, especially young women with the Type I Diabetes, who have unexplained poor blood glucose control and who lose nerve tissue cells. I would add measuring them for body fat and lean tissue as a technique to help them see what they are doing.

Insulin and Testing

Testing her blood glucose level several times daily helps Jan determine the amount of insulin to inject. The need to inject insulin was a major medical discovery, since enzymes and chemicals in the stomach and intestinal tract destroy insulin in pill form. The amount of insulin needed each day is determined by testing the amount of glucose in the blood, usually after waking, before lunch, dinner, and bedtime (See Chapter Notes). Sometimes blood glucose tests high for some unknown reason. Jan knew from previously testing her blood glucose, that some substances trigger a sudden rise in her blood glucose, so she consumes them sparingly (See Chapter Notes). She knows how exercise affected her blood glucose. She now eats before and after exercise. She was puzzled about the high blood glucose when she woke in the morning, a condition called the "Somogyi Effect" (See Chapter Notes). She thought she needed to increase her insulin and reduce her food intake. However, the treatment is actually the opposite. She needed to increase her store of glycogen during the day to carry her through the night and reduce her insulin dosages (See Chapter Notes).

Every few months, Jan has another blood test, the glycosylated hemoglobin test. The glycosylated hemoglobin test evaluates how well she has controlled her blood glucose over the previous six weeks to two months (See Chapter Notes).

Exercise

Exercise can control weight better than eliminating food or omitting insulin. But it can never be substituted for insulin. People with Type I Diabetes need to exercise aerobically about thirty to forty minutes several times a week. This kind of exercise can control blood triglycerides, LDL cholesterol and increase HDL cholesterol. Improving these blood levels is especially effective if the exercise is undertaken after a meal or snack when the greatest number of glucose molecules are circulating in the blood stream.

Exercising after eating also can prevent glucose from dropping below the normal range, which can occur if diabetics do not eat enough calories, exercise sporadically, too intensely or too long. Drinking water and eating a snack during exercise and then consuming, within thirty minutes after exercising about 10 to 15 grams of carbohydrate (a slice of bread) and some protein (1/2 cup of milk) may prevent blood glucose from dropping too low. This snack also can replace some of the glycogen and amino acids consumed by the muscle and liver cells during exercise.

The kind of exercise should be steady and rhythmic and use large muscles (legs and arms). As the muscles move, they absorb glucose molecules, oxygen, protein, and free fatty acids from the blood. The lungs bring in more oxygen to burn up the fatty acids in the blood. And for hours after the exercise, the rate increases at which all cells work. The muscles are stimulated to add more cells and become larger. The more muscle cells there are, the more glucose that can be absorbed from the blood, the less insulin that is needed and the less fat that is deposited.

Eliminate

For years, many people called blood glucose "blood sugar," and mistakenly believe that if "blood sugar" is low, they should eat sugar to replenish it. Because of this misinterpretation, I prefer that blood *glucose* be called just that, not "blood sugar." If the number of glucose molecules do drop below the normal range in the blood, a better solution than consuming some sugar is a glass of real fruit juice. Real fruit juice not only increases the number of glucose molecules fast but it contains some potassium and magnesium which can restore the integrity of lean tissue cells, something not possible with sugar or sugar substitutes.

Blood glucose may at some time drop so low that the person slips into a coma. Then sugar granules placed on their tongue would be appropriate or what would be better is an injection of glucagon. Both sugar and the glucagon are used to restore consciousness. Until their blood glucose is tested, sugar is far less dangerous than giving the person an injection of insulin.

Sugar substitutes and caffeine cannot replace sugar to restore a person's consciousness since they have no calories. Type I Diabetes, like those with Type II Diabetes, should avoid—better still, eliminate—sugar, alcohol, vitamin C and niacin supplements, and medications that raise blood glucose (See Chapter Notes). A high amount of sodium added to foods can also raise blood glucose. Therefore, eating foods as close to their natural state is always a better choice than eating processed foods.

By following the DIEET program and having the support of their family, doctor, nurse and registered dietitian, a person with Type I Diabetes can lead a normal and healthy life.

Pregnancy and Type I Diabetes

It is possible for women with Type I Diabetes to have a normal pregnancy and give birth to healthy children, contrary to what they may have heard. Judy had a successful pregnancy. She carefully planned for her pregnancy by preparing her body. She tightly controlled her blood glucose levels for several months before and then relied on a glycosylated hemoglobin blood test to tell her when conception was safe (See Chapter Notes). During her pregnancy, she again maintained a tight control over her blood glucose levels. She followed the DIEET program and the advice of her obstetrician.

During pregnancy there are many bodily changes. More estrogen is produced. Estrogen stimulates the liver to produce more glucose. More glucose requires more insulin. The demand for insulin increases as much as threefold over the non-pregnant state until it crescendos in the last three months. Therefore, to know how much insulin to inject, the woman needs to test her blood glucose several times a day. She needs to be sure she is eating her vegetables because the increase in insulin means more vitamin B6 is needed. Otherwise without the vitamin B6, the body produces a substance that inhibits insulin's action. Ingesting supplements can produce side effects in her and her fetus' body (See Chapter Notes for sources of vitamin B6 and Chapter 10 for toxicity levels).

The extra glucose, insulin and protein are needed to build the fetus' and mother's physical support system. The support system includes additional blood vessels that expands by one-third during pregnancy and an incubator (enlarged uterus and amniotic sac) for the fetus. Feeding this support system and the fetus requires an additional 300 calories a day or a total of 2300 to 2600 calories. A growing teenage girl, however, will need more—an extra 500 calories for a total of 2800 to 2900 calories. If the body doesn't receive the extra calories, then lean tissue will be converted to glucose and the by-products can pollute the blood and damage the fetus (See Chapter Notes).

What the pregnant woman puts in her mouth affects not only herself but the fetus. Abusive drugs and substances damage the fetus especially in the first few months of the pregnancy when foundation cells and the DNA for each cell are forming. Damaged cells can saddle the child with problems throughout life.

However, with preparation and careful monitoring of blood glucose during pregnancy, women with Type I Diabetes can deliver healthier babies than women who do not monitor, or feed themselves as well.

Children and Diabetes

Children with diabetes have different needs than adults. They are growing. Adults are not.

Carrie, a chubby 14-year-old with 18 percent body fat developed insulin-dependent diabetes. I designed a 1400-calorie meal plan of which 40 percent was fat. I weighed and measured her height and then measured her for body fat and lean tissue. In three months, she dropped eight pounds but 3 pounds were lean tissue and her blood glucose levels rose. She should have gained lean tissue because she was still growing.

The drop in lean tissue cells signaled to me that I had overly restricted her calories. So I increased them to 1800. When Carrie didn't gain any lean tissue weight and her blood glucose levels remained high, I increased her calories again . . . to 2000. We felt Carrie's body was receiving enough calories when her blood glucose stabilized. Her mother tracked her blood glucose and insulin doses. As she kept growing and adding lean tissue weight, I increased the calories until they peaked at 2600. As she grew, she lost body fat until it leveled off at 14 percent. She began menstruating at age 15, an indication she was approaching adulthood and would soon stop growing. At age 16, her lean tissue and height-stabilized so I reduced her caloric intake to 2200 with her daily fat calories set at 30 percent. Her blood glucose levels have remained within normal range and she has not been hospitalized in more than four years.

Her success and acceptance of her condition I believe stem from the relationship she has with her mother, a woman who encourages and praises her for following the DIEET program, for testing her own blood glucose, and who walks with her two to three miles every day. Carrie has developed into a beautiful young woman, with glowing skin, shiny hair, and beautiful teeth. She has a good self image and radiates happiness.

One in 600 school-age children usually develop Type I Diabetes, usually between the ages of six and eleven. As with diabetic adults, diabetic children can follow the DIEET guidelines: But with children, there are some differences. First, children are adding 200,000 lean tissue cells per minute and therefore as their lean tissue increases, so must the calories. How much can be determined by measuring and weighing the child each month. Examples are two 13-year-olds—a girl and a boy. She will need at least 2200 calories while he will need as much as 5000 calories. The amount depends on their activity output, their growth rate, their glycosylated hemoglobin levels and insulin needs (See Chapter Notes for calories).

Because of their smaller organs, children with diabetes need a slightly different combination of nutrients than adults. Carbohydrates are reduced to 48 to 50 percent of the calories to accommodate their small stomachs and intestinal tracts, fat is increased to 35 to 40 percent to reduce the load of carbon dioxide on their small lungs and protein is reduced to 12 percent of the calories to reduce the load of waste products on their small kidneys.

Overweight and obese children may have Type II Diabetes. A three hour glucose tolerance test can detect it and if so they should be started on the DEET program. Whether they are overweight or obese, they are growing. Obese girls need no less than 2,000 calories daily while obese boys, no less than 2400.

Substances such as sugar and caffeine, which interfere with blood glucose control are discouraged as are artificial sweeteners, particularly aspartame. The amino acids in aspartame may overwhelm a child's developing enzyme system and artificial sweeteners contain none of the nutrients necessary for a child's growth. Instead of sugar and artificial sweeteners, fruits and fruit juices can be incorporated into cookies, muffins, syrups, and beverages (See recipes in appendix).

 Exercise helps children control their blood glucose. It should be fun, rewarding, and accessible daily. Adequate food intake before exercise may be necessary to prevent blood glucose from sinking too low. A snack composed of a starch and a small amount of protein such as cereal and a cup of whole or two percent milk or a half sandwich of real cheese can prevent hypoglycemia.

Adapting to Being Diabetic

Many preteens and teens who have diabetes are afraid when they gain weight that they are becoming fatter. Convincing them to consume the recommended calories may take some innovative methods. There are several methods that I use to gain their trust. I measure them for their body fat and lean tissue weight each month, use a rubber band to show how they will stretch out and use "before and after" pictures. They and their parents need encouragement and praise for each step they take toward following the DIEET and DEET programs.

Children with diabetes may find themselves at odds with other children. If the child is made to feel different, he or she may take advantage of others and use their diabetic condition to manipulate others to get their way. Of course, a lot depends on the attitude of parents and siblings and the trust and rapport that the physician, dietitian, and nurse establish with the child and the family. Actually, entire families can embrace and receive benefit from the diabetic diet and exercise regime and prevent friction within the family. Children with diabetes will no doubt find themselves in situations where food is tempting. To help them, parents and dietitians can help them "role play" different food situations and provide words to say to those who offer them the tempting food.

Other help can come from support groups. A group of mothers, whose children had diabetes, and I organized a support group several years ago. Just before Halloween, the children were asked how they would handle "trick or treat." They had some very clever ideas. One monetary minded child said he would tell the people that he had diabetes and could not have candy, but he liked pennies. Another child would trade his candy with his friends for toys. Yet another would sell his candy to his parents and then buy something at the toy store. Their parents said they would hand out stickers, pencils, peanuts, little toys, plastic spiders or jewelry from the treasure box, crayons, and little comic books.

School parties can be a problem. Mothers said they discussed this with the teachers. They learned in advance what food would be served and then provided similar ones for their child: real juice versus KoolAid, graham crackers versus cookies, muffins versus cupcakes. Through trial and error, exchange of ideas with other parents and encouragement from the dietitian and physician, the parents and children learn that a regular schedule for testing blood, insulin injections, meals, snacks and sleep work best in controlling blood glucose. The body loves a rhythmic schedule, whether it is in a diabetic state or not.

I have asked several children and teenagers with diabetes if they consider themselves disadvantaged. They said they have accepted their diabetes, established a routine, feel good about their ability to control it and feel they are healthier than most other people their age. This is a salute to their parents who helped them learn, at a young age, to care for themselves and to be active participants in their own health. Similar results have been reported by the Joslin Clinic[21] which found that children with diabetes who were not forced to depend on the doctor, nurse, dietitian or their parents except in emergencies had developed a good self image. A foundation for health laid in their childhood can help children live a long life, with few complications of nerves, kidney damage, or heart disease.

Chapter Notes:

1: The three hormones which control blood glucose are produced in glands. The beta cells which produce insulin and the alpha cells which produce glucagon are in the pancreas. Cells which produce adrenaline are in adrenal gland. Insulin is needed to carry glucose and amino acids into the cells.

2: Building glycogen in the first two to two and a half hours after eating, glucose which is converted from food enters the blood stream and is distributed to the cells. Some of the cells receiving the glucose are the liver and muscle cells. They store the glucose as glycogen (up to 400 calories worth in the liver). The glycogen in the liver is used to provide glucose between meals but is depleted in about five or six hours (Muscle glycogen is not used to replace blood glucose). At about five hours after the meal, blood glucose drops signaling the hypothalamus hormone to send a hunger signal to the brain. If the person eats another well balanced meal with 600 to 900 calories and enough starches, the fuel cycle begins anew. Starches are the key and must be in bountiful amounts—360 to 540 calories each meal—because they convert 100 percent to glucose in the intestinal tract. That's more than can be said for protein or fat. Both of the latter are needed by the cells for their nutrients and calories but in much smaller quantities.

3: Foods that supply sufficient quantities of vitamin B6 are meat, fish or chicken, bananas, watermelon, baked potatoes, and green leafy vegetables. Foods that supply sufficient zinc are foods with high protein content such as meats, chicken, fish, seafood, turkey, eggs, venison, etc. Also wheat germ and wheat bran. Foods that contain sufficient chromium are liver, brewer's yeast, whole grains, nuts and cheese. Supplement form is not recommended.

4: To challenge insulin's release, blood should be drawn two hours after a meal. The person is instructed to consume a high carbohydrate diet for three consecutive days prior to testing. A postprandial blood glucose test normally should be less than 145 mg/dL. More than 160 mg/dL indicates a diabetic state. Additional blood tests that are used to detect Type II Diabetes are a cholesterol profile, a glycosylated hemoglobin and insulin (See Chapter Notes).

5: Statistics in 1987 revealed that 24 percent of adult men and 27 percent of adult women are considered overweight or obese, an increase of 40 percent since 1970. The definition for overweight is 10 percent over normal weight while obesity is 20 percent. A person whose normal weight is 120 pounds is overweight at 132 pounds and obese at 144 pounds. Of the people who are 10 percent overweight more are over 40 years of age 60 percent are men and 40 percent are women. The number of children who are overweight is 54 percent higher in ages 6 to 11 years and 39 percent higher in ages 12 to 18 than it was in 1963.

6: Hypoglycemic medications are: glipizide "Glucotrol," and glyburide "Glynase" and "Micronase."

7: Medications that raise blood glucose are contraceptive pills and estrogen, diuretics, prednisone, beta blockers, cortisone, testosterone, salicylates in large doses, and diphenylhydantoin (anti seizure medication). Propranolol (Inderal) raises blood glucose in those with Type II Diabetes, but reduces it in Type I Diabetes because propranolol enhances insulin secretion.

8: Anti-hypertensive medications that do not raise blood glucose are calcium channel blockers and angiotension converting enzyme inhibitors.

9: What happens if the hunger signal is ignored and the person chooses not to eat or eats no starch, or drinks diet pop or coffee or eats too few calories? Blood glucose drops further. Hypoglycemia sets in. Now the cells are without fuel and send off warning signs—like headaches. Others are tremors, chills, heart palpitations, numbness in the hands, feet, spaciness, weakness, sweating, hunger pangs, or irritability. These symptoms may be ignored and the person may complain to a doctor or take an over-the-counter medication to alleviate the misery. It may not seem apparent to them that they lack food. Without replenishing glucose with foods, lean tissue (and a little fat) are converted to glucose in an unsuccessful attempt by the liver to meet the cells' glucose demands. When the person finally eats, dietary glucose first is used to replace the fat and part of the lean tissue. Restoring the body's glycogen reserves is secondary.

10: Substances to eliminate are sugar, artificial sweeteners, alcohol, caffeine, vitamin C and niacin supplements, and medications that stimulate glucose to rise. The American Diabetes Association considers caffeine, tea, and sugar substitutes as free foods because they have no calories. This information is reiterated in health facilities. But calories are not the problem here. It is what happens after these substances enter the body and the way they affect the hormones. *They trigger a large release of insulin.* Many people believe they can just "have a little taste of dessert" or eat a small portion with few calories. But even a *smidgen* can send the glucose soaring, and the insulin pouring forth. Recovering from even a little indiscretion can set one back. Interestingly, dietary fat does not turn on the insulin hormone unless it is accompanied by sugar—as in chocolate candy, ice cream, or pastry, to name a few.

11: When a woman has gestational diabetes, she needs to inject insulin because her beta cells cannot produce enough insulin. The amount is determined by testing her urine and blood several times a day. Her goal is to keep her urine and blood free of ketones and her blood glucose below 150 mg/dL. The ketones damage the nerve and brain cells of the fetus.

12: In Type I Diabetes, the pancreas can lose its ability to produce enough insulin for several reasons. A genetic predisposition, when combined with environmental factors and a virus infection, can result in the destruction of specific cells. Susceptibility to diabetes increases four to ten times with a family predisposition. A virus can cause the immune system to produce antibodies that destroy the beta cells, particularly if they are genetically weak. A weak immune system cannot fight off a virus, cancer, or some other disease as well as a strong one. It can be weakened by dietary neglect, or if Type I Diabetes is not under control.

13: Symptoms of diabetes are: high blood pressure, urinary tract infections, vaginal infections, periodontal disease, menstrual irregularities, persistent fungal infections, and brown freckled shin spots.

14: Keeping blood glucose consistently between 90-110 mg/dL hinges not only on hormonal interactions but on how well the liver stores glycogen—an important source of fuel between meals. *The amount of glycogen stored depends not only on the amount of food eaten but also on the kind, consistency, and timeliness with which it is eaten.* Timing means putting fuel in the body before the person is active, something many people *automatically* consider for their cars, but not necessarily for themselves. The body machinery, shortly after arising heeds enough fuel to provide energy for the next five hours and every five hours after that. Remember every single minute the body needs two to three calories from food. This calculates out to 600-900 calories for each meal. Sometimes, blood glucose is high in the morning because of "Somogyl Effect" and not because the person had too much food, in fact, it's the opposite. Either the person did not consume enough food during the day to build up glycogen reserves to carry them through the night, or too much insulin was injected. Either way, during the night, blood glucose dropped. The adrenals and glucagon hormones respond and stimulate the liver to produce glucose. Too much glucose is dumped into the blood stream and by morning blood glucose is high. To build up the glycogen reserves, they can eat a snack mid-morning and mid afternoon or before bedtime and/or add one more starch and a fat at each meal. A suggestion for a snack is a peanut butter sandwich and fruit juice or 1/2 cup of milk.

15: There are several programs for people with Diabetes. I prefer to use what I call the "DEET" and "DIEET" programs, a modified version of the former "DIET" program.

16: The 2400 calories that most pregnant women consume are divided between 50-60 percent in carbohydrate, slightly lower in protein—12-15 percent, and slightly higher in fat—25-38 percent (See meal plans in Appendix)

17: The Recommended Dietary Allowances for children recommends that girls ages 10 to 12 years, whether diabetic or not, need 60 calories per kilogram of body weight or a total of 2300 calories daily. By the time girls are 15 years of age, growth slows and they need less calories per kilogram of body weight—45, or 2200 calories. Boys need more calories. They usually have more muscle and grow over a longer period of time than girls and usually have less body fat insulation. Boys aged 11 to 14 need, on the average, 2500 calories a daily. When boys reach 15 to 18 years of age, they need at least 3000. If they grow very fast in one year, they may need as many as 5000 calories. With exercise, this can reach a total of 7000 calories. These calories are divided into 38 percent fat, 12 percent protein, and 50 percent carbohydrates.

CHAPTER 7

Hypoglycemia
The Fuel Tank Registers Empty

HAS the following ever happened to you?

- You don't feel like eating breakfast and yet you should be hungry after eating for eight hours.

- You are nauseated in the morning.

- Suddenly you are exhausted, you can't take another step.

- You have a terrible headache.

- You can't stand the light or any noise.

- You are dizzy and tired in the afternoon.

- You have insomnia, sleep a few hours then you awaken and cannot get back to sleep.

- You have high blood cholesterol or heart arrythmias but cutting down on dietary fat, caffeine and nicotine hasn't helped.

- Your child has difficulty following directions. He is disruptive or hyperactive much of the day.

- Your best friend is high one minute and depressed the next.

- You've often wondered why alcoholics black out.

- You are a woman and wonder why you have cravings at certain times of the month.

What is Hypoglycemia?

Did you ever think that these signs and symptoms might be caused by hypoglycemia or low blood glucose? Hypoglycemia is defined in the *Dictionary of Medical Practice* as a deficiency of glucose in the blood stream. It is a condition rather than a disease.[22]

No organ, hormone, or enzyme escapes the damage of low blood glucose, especially if it is long term. Recognizing hypoglycemia is difficult because the symptoms may be mistaken for some other condition: nausea and headaches, to name two (See Chapter Notes). Hypoglycemia often accompanies diseases.

Because of the difficulty in distinguishing diseases and illnesses from hypoglycemia, many adults and children visit doctor after doctor seeking solutions to their disabling symptoms. Hypoglycemia became a popular subject of many books and magazine articles. Many attributed nearly every symptom a person experiences to it. Many people self diagnose themselves and seek help from over-the-counter medications, herbs, and vitamin and mineral supplements. Hypoglycemia can be a serious condition with serious consequences to oneself and to others, if not diagnosed and treated.

I talked with a woman who didn't realize the seriousness of hypoglycemia. She told me she was driving into town one day when suddenly, she passed out and her car hit an abutment. Fortunately, her car was the only one involved and she was not badly injured. She said she had experienced momentary blackout episodes before, but she was at home where she could immediately eat. She decided to seek help after her close call.

To diagnose true hypoglycemia, people with the symptoms should have a glucose tolerance test. This will reveal whether they have diabetes, reactive hypoglycemia, or fasting hypoglycemia (See Chapter Notes). However, the five hour glucose tolerance test must be supervised by a physician since the test itself can be dangerous. Fasting hypoglycemia, a rare occurrence, is so serious it can lead to coma and death unless it is treated.

Reactive Hypoglycemia

A more common occurrence is reactive hypoglycemia. Reactive hypoglycemia can range from mild and tolerant to serious and disabling. Most people experience the mild hypoglycemia but, because it is so transient and passes so quickly, they are unaware of it. However, if someone has the more serious kind they are very aware that something is wrong. The episode may begin with over-exercising, or when a severe reducing diet is followed. The type of hypoglycemia that scares people suddenly starts about two to four hours after they have eaten a meal. Movement and speaking may be restricted even though sight and hearing are not. The timing appears to coincide with the "switchover" between hormones as blood glucose drops below normal. The nerves signal the pancreas to release glucagon and raise blood glucose. Ordinarily, blood glucose rises immediately. But with hypoglycemia, the process can take longer. The responding hormones like glucagon, are too sluggish, allowing too much lag time. The lag time leaves symptoms for 24 hours after blood glucose has returned to normal.

Many people find that they can eat something and feel better. Feeding yourself after the attack is somewhat like driving the car into the garage after the hail storm hits. The damage has been done. Without glucose and oxygen, brain cells can starve, suffocate and die and, if the hypoglycemia lasts, as it does with lag time, can result in permanent damage because the brain only has enough glucose to last a few minutes. Recognizing a signal *before* blood glucose drops can allow you time to feed yourself and thus prevent the loss of brain cells. Time is of the essence. One signal is a yawn. A yawn indicates a drop in the oxygen level in the brain, a reflection also of a drop in blood glucose. Glucose, the source of energy, must be present for the brain to absorb oxygen.

Lack of Sleep

Another sign of hypoglycemia is interrupted sleep. People usually tell me that they can't sleep because they have too much on their minds. True, anxiety, stress, pain, and unnerving experiences can prevent sleep. All of these affect the hormones which control blood glucose. Lack of sleep may not be identified as hypoglycemia in the true sense of the word, but the brain is the first organ to be affected by a drop in blood glucose.

What helps you sleep soundly and experience less pain is the neurotransmitter, serotonin. Serotonin is a substance that the brain produces from tryptophan and cholesterol with the help of vitamin B6. Tryptophan is an essential amino acid from foods such as meat, eggs, fish, poultry and milk products.

There is a catch. The brain must have plenty of glucose from starchy foods and from the glycogen stored in the liver for tryptophan to make serotonin. Often people use sleep medications and a few years ago they bought the tryptophan supplement. But the government removed the supplements from the market when they were linked to several deaths. Sleep medications may help by affecting the brain but they do not restore liver glycogen. The lack of serotonin also results in aggressive behavior and thoughts of suicide.

When people awaken during the night and cannot get back to sleep, it can be a sign that the liver has run out of its storage of glycogen and has begun converting protein in lean tissue to glucose. This protein includes tryptophan. Not only has tryptophan been lost from some cells, but the production of glucose from lean tissue is too slow and blood glucose drops.

As a safer alternative to sleeping medications, I've suggested the following: Go to the kitchen and eat a snack consisting of some starch and some protein such as cheese or milk *and* crackers or bread *and* drink some warm liquid. This usually works.

At the same, I encourage people to consume enough calories and nutrients at each of three meals (600 to 700) and a snack *during* the day to build up their glycogen stores and also to bypass substances such as caffeine, alcohol, nicotine and artificial sweeteners which prevent the storage of glycogen (See Chapter Notes).

Women may notice that just before their menstrual period they have more trouble sleeping and crave food, especially sweets. They are experiencing "hypoglycemia." The brain senses the drop in blood glucose and sends a message to the hypothalamus for the person to eat, triggering a craving for sweets.

Alcohol is sneaky because it triggers sleepiness. But after a few hours, people awaken with insomnia. The problem again: the body's source of glucose. The liver can store or convert very little glycogen while it is detoxifying alcohol. The alcohol itself, although it has calories, provides no glycogen. Additionally, alcohol dehydrogenase uses up vitamin B6, the very nutrient needed to convert tryptophan to serotonin. Alcohol irritates other cells, such as the hormones which regulate blood glucose.

As a stimulant, caffeine itself can affect sleep because it stimulates the nerves. Caffine supplies no glycogen and depletes the glycogen that is stored. By late afternoon, you may become very tired. Uninterrupted sleep will be difficult.

Sugar and Hypoglycemia

Sugar creates similar problems. It is digested so fast that the liver is overwhelmed and cannot convert it all to glycogen. So most of it is converted to fat. In about 15 or 30 minutes, blood glucose drops. Frequent ingestion of sugar and caffeine effects the hormones that regulate blood glucose. When the hormones must respond many times a day to sugar and caffeine, year in and year out, they can eventually become sluggish or overactive. If the beta cells become overactive, they can over secrete insulin, driving glucose to abnormally low levels within two or three hours after a meal.

Some children eat sugar and become hyperactive or disruptive or both. Others do not, perhaps because they have more mature systems. The children who are hyperactive or disruptive are often labeled with Attention Deficit Disorder. Usually, a medication is prescribed. But the children may never have had the benefit of dietary analysis or a glucose tolerance test.

Herrick, three years old, could have been a candidate for medication if he had not had a glucose tolerance test.

Herrick would not sleep. His mother was desperate. Her husband gave her an ultimatum. He would have to sleep elsewhere if she did not control their son. Her husband was exhausted because their three year old son was in and out of their bed every night and was disruptive during the day. The mother took Herrick to several doctors who conducted various brain wave tests or put him in the hospital for other studies. The doctors were puzzled. Everything was normal.

The mother took Herrick to my husband, a pediatrician, who ordered a three hour oral glucose tolerance test. By the second hour, Herrick's blood glucose had dropped precipitously. The doctor terminated the test and referred Herrick's parents to me.

The parents told me that they were so distraught that they even gave their son some beer before bedtime but it did not help him sleep. His disruptiveness led the nursery school director to ask for his removal from school.

I provided a meal plan for Herrick but admonished the parents not to give him any beer, caffeine, sugar, fructose, syrup, honey, molasses, or dextrose. I showed them how to read the ingredients on product labels. The following week they were all smiles. At the end of Herrick's first full day without any sugar and with fairly good meals, the parents put their child to bed. They checked on him before retiring. He was asleep. The next morning they awoke with a start. Their child had not been in their bedroom all night. He was still sleeping in his room, the first full night's sleep he had had in more than a year.

Two months later, the nursery school director agreed to the mother's request that if the boy was no longer disruptive, he could return to school. But before the interview for re-admission, the director placed everything high up on the shelves. However, it wasn't necessary. Herrick played quietly with his toys. The director asked what medication he was on. The mother told her he was on none adding that she had eliminated sugar from her son's diet. The director thought the other parents could benefit from this experience. During the meeting, one woman who sat in the front row cried. She said a similar thing has happened to her, but her husband divorced her. She did not know about sugar's effect on behavior.

It is possible that Herrick could not sleep because he was eating sugar, but more importantly he was depleting his body of nutrients.

Seizures

Low blood glucose affects the developing brain differently than a developed brain. The adult brain has a few minutes worth of glucose, but a child's brain has less. Newborns have even less than an older child. Physicians treating newborns know that the newborn will suffer serious brain damage from hypoglycemia unless treated promptly. Because they have less capacity to store glucose, children have more of a tendency to have seizures when blood glucose drops precipitously than adults do. Seizures can occur in susceptible children after they have gone too long without food, exercised too much, ingested offending substances such as alcohol in cough syrup, (See Chapter Notes) have lead poisoning, suffered trauma to the brain, have a congenital disorder or an error of metabolism.

During a seizure, the body uses a great deal more calories, glucose, and nutrients to supply the energy for the excess firing of neurons. Normally, the brain alone uses about 400 to 500 calories a day. But with all the energy used by the neurons, less is available for the rest of the body, including the brain. After a seizure, people usually go limp and fall asleep. Because the glucose is diverted each time a person has a seizure, the brain and nerves suffer more damage.

It makes sense then, to prevent seizures. And to prevent seizures, hypoglycemia must be averted. To prevent hypoglycemia, calories with nutrients need to be consumed more often during the day, most likely every two to two and one-half hours. A snack in the middle of the night may also be necessary. The meals should be high in fat—about 40 to 43 percent for children—for several reasons. The most important is to provide calories. The second reason is to slow the transit time as the food passes through the intestinal tract. This slower time allows the glucose to enter the blood stream continually over several hours, maintaining a more normal blood glucose (See Chapter Notes). Sugars, alcohol, and caffeine can spike a rise and then a drop in blood glucose. An example involves the story about one of my patients and his mother.

Many years ago a woman telephoned seeking a diet to control her 12-year-old son's seizures. I provided the youth with a meal plan containing enough calories to cover his lean tissue and growth. The amount of protein I allotted was 12 percent and the fat content was 35 percent. He was to eat every three to four hours. The plan also included the elimination of sugar, caffeine, alcohol, sugar substitutes, and monosodium glutamate, but I admonished her to continue the prescribed medication.

She telephoned me nine years later to ask if I could help her son again. She told me that she was originally motivated to follow the meal plan because she did not want to give her son a lot of medication. She baked her own bread and grew and canned her own vegetables and fruits. She also eliminated the substances I recommended. She was proud to report that he had not had a single seizure in nine years. She was calling me now because he had had three seizures in three months. He had recently married and was reluctant to criticize his bride's cooking. I told her I thought she was the best teacher, but that I would help if needed.

Some children with seizures have been helped with the ketogenic diet in which the dietary fat in a meal is much higher than 40 percent. But for this diet the children need to be closely supervised in a hospital first and the parents need to receive instructions on how to feed and monitor their child at home.

Hyperactivity

Not all children with hypoglycemia have seizures but they have other symptoms. The symptoms are poor attention span and concentration, hyperactivity, disruptiveness, and inability to follow directions. To control these symptoms, hypoglycemia must be prevented. The children will need to be treated nutritionally just like those subject to seizures (See Chapter Notes). Otherwise the hypoglycemia and behavior may escalate.

Roger, a nine year old boy, was extremely disruptive and could not concentrate in school. He often had to be reprimanded; he hit other children and interrupted the teacher. He had no friends. His parents consulted a pediatrician whose examination found him to be healthy. However, a four-hour oral glucose tolerance test revealed hypoglycemia. When he was referred to me, I provided his parents with a meal plan for him with enough calories and nutrients to allow for his growth; I asked him to eliminate the sugar. His sister said "He has a lollipop in his pocket." I said, "I think Roger will give it up when he is ready." He handed it to me as he started out the door. That first week he tried very hard not to have any candy or sugar. The only episode occurred when he mistook fruit drink for fruit juice at a birthday party. But he was very proud of himself. He had refused the ice cream and cake. His teacher commented how well he behaved in school. A few weeks later he joined a softball team and proudly told me that he had a friend.

Changes in Personality

When the brain is subjected to repeated episodes of glucose deficiency, changes occur in personality and intellectual ability resulting in psychotic or bizarre behavior or outbursts of temper. Energy needs rise with each outburst of temper, anxiety and over-excitedness, tension and stress. Blood pressure rises, the pulse quickens, the skin reddens, the muscles strain. All of this takes as much energy as a seizure. The adrenal glands react and blood glucose rises. Insulin pours forth. But soon blood glucose plunges into hypoglycemia. The person perspires, feels weak and faint, has heart palpitations and loses his or her appetite. The stomach produces excess acid. Food that had been eaten earlier moves through the intestinal tract too quickly for digestion. The intestinal tract reacts with nausea, vomiting, diarrhea and/or an irritable colon. Signaling of low blood glucose.

Often these mental and personality changes are misdiagnosed, especially in the young and the elderly.

Hypoglycemia may be manifested in children through their stomach and intestinal tracts. They may react to their environment or to television programs which frighten them. An upset child is more vulnerable to hypoglycemia.

Hypoglycemia can be prevented if you anticipate an emotional problem and forestall it by feeding yourself or the other person beforehand. Stress is always handled better when you have a full stomach. We had a saying in our house, "Never approach your father about a problem until he has eaten." So our children would ask him, "Have you had your supper?" "Yes." "Okay, then you can look at my report card."

Offending Substances

Many people have had hypoglycemia for years and live with it until it becomes disabling. But "living with it" can negatively affect a person's health. Such was the case of Katie.

Katie had been given eight injections and several medications to help her become pregnant. She had been ingesting vitamin supplements since childhood. When she became pregnant she added the maternal supplements. After giving birth, she restricted her calories to lose excess weight. She said that whether she was pregnant or not, she had endured diarrhea or constipation, gas, and bloating for years.

She came to see me because she had heard that diet could help hypoglycemia. Hypoglycemia attacks were no stranger to her. She had experienced attacks which left her weak, shaky, nauseated, and sweaty. Her fingers and toes felt numb. If she ate, the symptoms faded. She told me she had been having these intermittent attacks for twelve years, during which time she married. But no other attack was like the two most recent ones. They scared her. Her baby was only a few months old when she had two sudden episodes that paralyzed her to the point that she could not call for help.

She said that during her pregnancy she was so nauseated that she couldn't eat and had stomach pains and diarrhea. Her doctor diagnosed hypoglycemia after her blood glucose levels dropped to 24 mg/dL, or 66 mg per 100 milliliters below normal, during a five-hour glucose tolerance test. She said he had suspected a tumor in her pancreas but tests ruled it out. His additional diagnosis: irritable bowel.

I suspected that her low calorie diet and the many vitamin supplements she was taking contributed to her irritable bowel and her severe hypoglycemic episodes. What effect the fertility drug had on Katie's hypoglycemia and intestinal tract is an unknown although the manufacturers list low blood glucose as a side effect. However, they do not address long term ramifications.

Katie and I set a goal and a plan. The goal was to repair the intestinal tract and to reduce the hypoglycemic symptoms with food. I provided her with a 2000 calorie daily meal plan which she was to divide into six or seven meals. I suggested she eliminate the vitamin supplements on a trial basis. She had already eliminated alcohol, cigarettes, and sugar.

As her intestinal tract repaired, the hypoglycemia waned and she lost weight. With her second pregnancy, I increased her calories to 2500, divided among six meals. She decided to eliminate the vitamin supplements. It was an easy pregnancy for her. Since then, she has had a few, less severe hypoglycemic episodes, but she can now pinpoint their cause.

Low blood glucose can result from medications, prescribed or over-the-counter or excessive doses of vitamin or mineral supplements which may interfere with the blood glucose regulatory process, or which affect the brain, the nerves or intestinal tract (See Chapter Notes).

Other medications may be able to steady blood glucose and improve the person's behavior. For instance, people can be diagnosed with panic and anxiety disorders, hyperactivity, and depression. But the underlying problem is not always addressed. If medications are prescribed, a diet history and diet can enhance the response just as it does when insulin is prescribed for diabetes.

Pre-diabetes

Hypoglycemia may be a sign of pre-diabetes, either Type I or Type II. Both diabetes and hypoglycemia involve blood "sugar" and have one thing in common, the hormone, insulin. *Hypo*glycemia, like *hyper*-glycemia, is a signal that blood glucose is not under control. In hypoglycemia, either the body has an excess of insulin which disposes of the glucose too quickly or the hormones that counter the drop in blood glucose do not react in a timely manner. Some people may think they should take chromium picolinate to improve their glucose regulating hormones, but there are no documented studies. Hypoglycemia is not to be taken lightly or treated with over the counter remedies. Hypoglycemia can do more harm in less time than the high blood glucose of diabetes.

Diseases and Hypoglycemia

Hypoglycemia can occur anytime there is a disorder involving an organ, or a disease that is not under control as can occur with diabetes. People taking medications for hypothyroidism can experience hypoglycemia if they forget to take their dosage or if they eat foods with goitrogens (cabbage, cauliflower, brussels sprouts, and broccoli). Goitrogens interfere with the work of the thyroid and thyroid medication (See Chapter Notes).

Heart arrhythmias or angina can often be a sign of low blood glucose. If a person has an auto-immune disease such as cancer, arthritis, lupus or multiple sclerosis, they may complain of being cold. Being cold often means they have low blood glucose because their body is not storing enough glycogen. Usually, people with these diseases do not have the appetite to consume enough calories and nutrients to keep up with the tremendous number their immune system uses to fight the disease.

Toxins and Hypoglycemia

A reaction to a toxin often signals low blood glucose. The body reacts to toxins entering the body more if the liver is not well fed and is not storing enough glycogen. Without enough energy the liver has less ability to detoxify toxins as they enter through the skin, lungs, or mouth especially as they age. The reaction to a toxin is not always a result of too few calories and nutrients. A strong toxin can overwhelm even a well fed liver. A toxin can be any substance touch, smell or taste (See Chapter Notes for other suspicious substances). The reaction leaves people feeling weak, lethargic or in pain. They may have a headache or difficulty breathing.

Alcohol

Alcohol can be a toxin, especially if consumed in excess. Drinking large amounts of alcohol is not always considered serious in our society. When a person drinks too much alcohol or drinks it too fast, the liver is too busy producing alcohol dehydrogenase to produce enough glucose causing them to experience hypoglycemia. When there is a lack of glucose a person has blurred vision, wobbly legs, and they can't speak or think clearly. Recovery from an alcohol hypoglycemic attack can be much slower if the person has been without food.

Tracking A Hypoglycemic Episode

If the person believe they have hypoglycemic episodes, I suggest that a diary be kept. In the diary they should note not only the exact time of the symptoms but what was eaten and any toxins that may have been encountered then action can be taken (See Appendix for sample).

The Care and Diet of People with Hypoglycemia

If someone suffers from the disabling effects of hypoglycemic episodes they should follow this special program. This program is designed to build up their glycogen storage but it is not a guarantee. What I hope is the program can help them improve their quality of life, increase their energy for work and play so that they can enjoy their family, friends, and home.

- **Meals**: Three (or six small ones) should be eaten daily plus a snack. The calories should be based on the calories needed to support the person's lean tissue. Since morning is a time when many people experience hypoglycemia, and the liver is deficient in glycogen, breakfast should be eaten even before the person dresses or exercises. Blood glucose normally drops about five hours after a meal, so try to eat before the five hours are up. However, if it is noticed that blood glucose drops in two and one half hours then the meal should be eaten every two and one half hours from breakfast on. Calories for each meal should be fairly even with about 600-700 for each of the three meals or 325 to 400 for each of the six meals. Adults need more carbohydrate and less fat than children (See Meal Plans in Appendix). Children need less protein (12 percent) and more fat (35-40). Sometimes a hypoglycemic attack comes while they are in a car, at work, school, or in a meeting. Should they eat the candy bar or lifesaver which is in their pocket or smoke a cigarette? Should they take the medication or the vitamin pill they bought at the drug store? Should they drive through a fast food restaurant for a coke or some coffee, or stop at a bar for a drink? These choices may make them feel better for a short period of time, but it won't last. The more prudent action is to plan ahead and carry extra food with them because they never know when a hypoglycemia attack will occur. Having the snack on hand can give them peace of mind knowing that they can prevent an attack. A combination of starch and a protein food maintains the blood glucose level longer than a starch alone (See Chapter Notes).

- **Offending substances**: The following should be eliminated because they can lead to hypoglycemia (See Chapter Notes): sugar, nicotine, caffeine, alcohol, vitamin and mineral supplements and medications whose side effects increase or decrease blood glucose (See Chapter Notes).

- **Liquid**: Drink two cups of water with each meal with a cup between meals. Water also should be drunk before exercise, every ten minutes during exercise, and when finished.

- **Sleep**: Adults should sleep eight hours; children 10 to 12.

- **Exercise**: People should exercise aerobically at a moderate level for 20 to 30 minutes but after a meal or snack. They may need to eat some starch food and a liquid within 15 minutes after finishing the exercise.

Summary

Even though hypoglycemia is not a disease, it should not be ignored. Some kinds of hypoglycemia can lead to brain damage. Repeated hypoglycemic episodes can produce erratic blood glucose levels which can create emotional havoc. The goal is to prevent these episodes. The body is never on vacation and needs the kind of fuel as well as enough fuel every five hours which will protect the lean tissue cells. The treatment may be as simple as excluding some substances that precipitate the rise in blood glucose. Or it may be as simple as following a program that is similar to the one for those with diabetes. A high protein, low carbohydrate diet does not work for those with diabetes, and it does not work for those with hypoglycemia.

Chapter Notes:

1: Other symptoms of hypoglycemia are: mood swings, hunger pangs, uncontrolled temper, perspiring palms, night sweats, disorientation, restlessness, weakness, unexplained waking in the night, inability to stay awake, impotency, frigidity, forgetfulness, low sex drive, and sudden phobias. Body temperature may fall to 96 degrees; the person may feel cold in a house heated between 80 and 85 degrees.

2: Hypoglycemia may be caused by a substance in the diet, from skipping meals, too few calories, or too little fat in the meals. It can be caused by a surplus of vitamins or minerals in supplement form, or medications. It can be a result of an allergic reaction or some underlying disease. Other offending substances are sugar, caffeine, nicotine, alcohol, toxins, and medications which.

3: A meal with protein, fat, and complex carbohydrates eaten every five hours slows down the pace of digestion which then slows the number of glucose molecules entering the blood stream; this tempers the highs and lows of blood glucose.

4: Medications that can increase blood glucose are: salicylates (aspirin, Bufferin, Ascriptin, Ecotrin, Empirin) especially in infants and children. Other medications are: propranodol (Inderal), Haldol, Darvon, anti-histamines, and oxidase inhibitor drugs (Nardil) and isoniazid (an anti-tubercular drug).

5: Goitrogens prevent the absorption of iodine, the mineral necessary for the thyroid gland to produce hormone thyroxin. They are the cabbage family, cauliflower, Brussels sprouts rutabagas, and turnips. Large quantities of the following may act as goitrogens: peaches, almonds, soybeans and cassava, ground nuts and peanuts, and PABA (para-aminobenzoic acid), a vitamin-like substance.

6: Examples of toxins are: underarm deodorant and perfume, detergents and cleaning supplies, cosmetics and hair dye, cigarette smoke and exhaust from factories, chocolate and peanuts, potatoes and cinnamon.

CHAPTER 8

Breathless Without Fuel

IT is a clear gorgeous day with low humidity when you step outside and inhale a deep breath of fresh air. The oxygen travels straight to your toes, combusting with glucose from breakfast and you feel a surge of energy.

We take our breathing pretty much for granted until our lungs are damaged. Unconsciously, we inhale and exhale rhythmically 14 to 18 times a minute. Working every moment, 24 hours a day, the lungs never take a vacation and use a fair amount of glucose and nutrients. Because they constantly need energy, they are among the first to be affected when calories are scarce.

When oxygen is inhaled it travels to the cells where it joins glucose and combusts to energy resulting in two waste products—water and carbon dioxide. The water is excreted; the carbon dioxide exhaled.

Caution: Lungs At Work

There are two lungs. Each lung contains lobes; the right has three, the left has two. Each pair of lungs contains 750 million balloon-like air sacs that contain a material called elastin. The elastin is a protein which acts just like it sounds. It allows the air sacs to inflate when oxygen enters and to deflate when carbon dioxide leaves. Surrounding the air sacs are capillaries of blood that pick up the oxygen and carry it to all the cells. A cage of ribs protects the lungs. Below the lungs is a diaphragm that works similar to a bellows as a person breathes. Connecting the ribs and diaphragm to the muscles is connective tissue which is very flexible. Respiratory muscles respond involuntarily (See Chapter Notes).

As our lungs inhale, they are subjected to numerous pollutants, including dust, dirt, germs, and smoke. To prevent these pollutants from entering the rest of the body, the lungs produce enzymes which break down the pollutants into harmless particles. All this work by the lungs requires calories and nutrients on a regular basis.

When air sacs are damaged they rupture and join with other sacs to form larger ones. These larger sacs are more likely to trap carbon dioxide instead of releasing it. Gradually, the carbon dioxide builds up and replaces the incoming oxygen. Additionally, when the tiny blood vessels carrying the oxygen from the air sacs break down, less oxygen enters the blood stream. The result is bronchitis, pneumonia, progressing to emphysema. People gasp for air as if they were drowning. Only drowning is quicker.

Many conditions can precipitate this lack of oxygen. Genes and the lack of calories and nutrients are potent factors. An intestinal tract which compromises the body's supply of nutrients can also take a toll on the lungs. An overwhelming pollutant is a third (See Chapter Notes).

What happens to the lungs when the caloric intake is reduced, when meals are skipped or substituted with a candy bar, soft drink, coffee, or smoking a cigarette instead of eating? The protein in the lung cells, the elastin, the connective tissue, the tiny blood vessels and the air sacs can be recruited for glucose.

When Unloaded Fuel Becomes Loaded

As the cells dwindle in number, less working lung cells are available. But we hardly miss them in the beginning. We may notice we are more exhausted at the slightest exertion and may declare "I must be out of shape." It may begin with a respiratory infection, sinus trouble, asthma or pneumonia. The progression may be slow until one day breathing becomes difficult.

As breathing becomes more labored, muscle energy demands increase, creating a vicious cycle. With less cells to do the work of many, the respiratory muscles are overtaxed and underfed, their own protein and glycogen convert to glucose.

The more cells that are lost, the more malnourished they become and the more difficult it is for them to breathe which places more pressure on the lung lobes. Too much pressure can cause a lobe to collapse. As it continues, an ever tighter spiraling descent to malnutrition which begets emphysema and chronic lung disease.

Emphysema is a disease that slowly and permanently destroys the delicate air sacs in the lungs, leaving more carbon dioxide to damage them. The reduced lung power means more energy is required, and the person gasps for air.

The Effect of Carbon Dioxide on Lungs

An image of a person with emphysema may be someone who is thin, gaunt, emaciated, and malnourished. But overweight people can have chronic lung problems too. The thin people with emphysema are called "pink puffers" because their lungs are hyper inflated, their diaphragm stays flat and doesn't rise. Overweight people with breathing difficulty are called "blue bloaters" because as they retain more carbon dioxide, and gain water weight.

The more people struggle to breathe, the more calories they need, the more lean tissue weight they lose. Those with Chronic Obstructive Pulmonary Disease (COPD), underestimate the number of calories that their labored breathing requires. If they continue to lose weight, heart failure or cancer are in the offing (See Chapter Notes). The sooner they break the cycle of losing lean tissue weight, the less lung tissue they will lose and the more their lung function can improve.

One way to improve lung function is through diet. Fat produces four times less carbon dioxide than carbohydrates combust with oxygen. Therefore, we change the ratio of fat to carbohydrate, making them equal—43 percent of the calories (See Meal Plans in the Appendix).

This higher percent fat may seem feasible for the thin person who needs to gain weight, but for the overweight person? Reducing calories too much increases the risk of lung damage, resulting in more exhaustion and more accumulation of carbon dioxide, water and weight. The extra water and body fat press up against the diaphragm, preventing the lungs from inflating and deflating fully. Limiting the amount of oxygen inhaled and reducing the amount of carbon dioxide exhaled. Because of this constriction on their diaphragm, "blue bloaters" have difficulty losing weight.

Mary Anna was about 30 pounds overweight. She had been consulting with me for several weeks when, immediately after she arrived for an appointment one day, she asked to be weighed. Fifteen minutes later she asked to be weighed again. She had gained five pounds! She had consumed no food or drink. She was just breathing and talking.

Since this event occurred, several other people have told me that they can feel when they are "filling up" with water and when they step on the scales they have gained five to eight pounds within a short time. Normally, there are shifts of water in the body over a 24 hour period but these are not dramatic.

"Blue bloaters" typically develop bronchitis rather than emphysema and are not as malnourished as the "pink puffers."

Both "blue bloaters" and "pink puffers" need to exercise. First they need a pulmonary function test and then permission from their physician. When "blue bloaters" consume the high fat diet and exercise they surprisingly lose body fat and gain some lean tissue. They have more energy because they breathe with less exertion and they feel better; amazingly, their cholesterol remains normal. Actually, the extra fat helps the liver make cholesterol which the lungs need to make new cells.

Nicotine and Other Pollutants

It goes without saying that people with lung problems need clean air. Imagine the damage to the lungs when a pollutant such as tobacco smoke with its 30 plus carcinogenic substances and carbon monoxide are superimposed on a low calorie diet, and why lung destruction is so rapid. It has been reported that nicotine reduces lung capacity 50 percent faster than normal aging. Nicotine has the potential to destroy the quality and shorten the length of life. But oh so subtly! At least one research scientist claims that each time people smoke they lose five and one half minutes of their life, and over their life expectancy, five to eight years. Double that if they smoke and do not eat.

Why do people like to smoke so much? They might recite, "What else can give me a lift quickly, help me perform better, relieve my anxiety yet not make me gain weight?"

It is true. Nicotine stimulates the adrenal glands which signal the liver to release glucose giving the person a burst of energy and a calming effect. Temporarily smokers may see better, think more clearly, and feel relaxed. But this doesn't last. Soon they need another fix.

Many people who smoke don't have an appetite and therefore eat too few calories. 20 percent of smokers say they use this potent appetite suppressant to control their weight. What really happens is the nicotine destroys the nerve endings in the tongue and nose.

A problem with nicotine is the debris it leaves behind in the lung, reducing the lungs' capacity to inhale and exhale. Smoke destroys the nerve endings of the cilia cells as it passes through them (See Chapter Notes). The cilia protect the lungs from dust, germs, and bacteria. Without the cilia, the carcinogenic tars and carbon monoxide, cyanide and 30 other irritants in tobacco, adhere to and destroy the lung cells.

Nicotine is a poison. It kills bugs and people. Each cigarette contains two milligrams of nicotine. If a child eats two cigarettes or six cigarette butts, they can die.

As nicotine enters the blood, it reaches the brain in seven seconds and each cell in the body in 15 seconds. Each working cell must then process the nicotine and carbon monoxide with three antioxidants, vitamin C, vitamin A, and vitamin E or be damaged. Normally, the amount of vitamin C a person needs in a day is 60 mg which is enough for it to carry out its many jobs. It forms collagen, the protein part of connective tissue, It wards off infections by preventing the break down of cells by oxygen. When nicotine is present, the cells need twice as much vitamin C (See Chapter Notes).

Are Supplements the Answer?

Should you take a supplement? Supplements will provide the extra vitamin C, but they do not provide the macro nutrients needed to build the lung cells. Actually, a former smoker only needs to drink a glass of orange juice for five or six days to replace a deficiency in vitamin C.

As for vitamin E, the recommended amount of 10 to 15 I.U. is enough to protect the red and white blood cells which pass through the air sacs and is enough to prevent infections and many diseases. But when nicotine is present, the cells use vitamin E quickly, denying other cells their share. Smokers who eat a diet of white flour products, low- fat or fried foods develop a deficiency of vitamin E. Taking a vitamin E supplement may help in the beginning, but again it does not provide the needed macro-nutrients and, if taken over an extensive period, can cause thinning of the blood, bleeding, and/or hemorrhages. The solution is to eliminate the cigarettes and eat foods with vitamin E.

Vitamin A helps fight infections, keeps the mucous membranes healthy and prevents damage to the cilia. But, smoking irritates the mucous membranes which can result in lung, oral, bladder, kidney, pancreatic, cervical or esophageal cancer.

Women who smoke have a greater risk for osteoporosis than those who don't because smoking increases the rate of estrogen breakdown. Nicotine irritates the intestinal tract preventing digestion and interfering with cell repair in the lungs and elsewhere.

The Dangers of Carbon Monoxide

Tobacco contains another pollutant, carbon monoxide, which displaces oxygen and poisons the brain cells and all vital organs. Smokers' blood has two to 15 times more carbon monoxide than non-smokers' blood. The result is that the arteries harden. Red blood cells increase, blood thickens. The lining in the blood vessels shrink, taxing and enlarging the heart as it pumps the thicker blood through the smaller channels. Blood pressure and pulse rate rise. Blood vessels constrict and blood circulation is reduced. With less circulation, males become impotent, the skin, fingers, and toes become cold, eyes develop glaucoma. The lack of glucose and oxygen to the brain makes the smoker mentally tired and at risk for Alzheimer's disease.

Why Does Smoking Make One Lose Weight?

Outward signs of the loss of lean tissue cells from smoking cigarettes are yellow fingers and nails; premature wrinkling around the mouth, eyes, and throat; lack of taste and gravely voice. The premature wrinkling results from the lack of oxygen.

Another sign is the added body fat around the waist. Maybe smokers believe that nicotine helps them become or remain thin. It may, but the kind of weight they lose is lean tissue weight, as evidenced by their wasted buttocks. A better solution is to eliminate the smoking and to exercise.

Pregnancy and Smoking

It is common knowledge that nicotine affects the fetus of a pregnant woman. The fetus's brain receives less oxygen and therefore, the newborn is born underweight. An infant born into a household of smokers will have smaller lungs which may not be able to produce enough of the enzymes to break down the carbon monoxide and carbon dioxide of secondhand smoke. With less oxygen, infants are at risk for sudden infant death syndrome. Secondhand smoke causes infants and children to have more infections, colds, and earaches. Such infections can interfere with the children's growth and development and can damage their respiratory system for life. Passive smoking causes as many health problems as active smoking. Nonsmokers also absorb tar, carbon monoxide, and nicotine just as much as smokers do.

It is difficult to quit smoking. Weight gain may occur after someone quits but they will be gaining back some of the lost lean tissue which includes their lung cells, bone cells, blood vessels, etc. With exercise they can increase their lean tissue even more, burn up body fat, remain thin and become healthier than when they smoked.

Other Pollutants

Nicotine is but one pollutant which displaces oxygen and damages lung tissue. Ozone is another. Ozone forms when automobiles, busses, and airplanes emit nitrogen oxide and hydrocarbons. When mixed with sunlight and humidity, ozone rises and oxygen availability falls. Other pollutants are: chlorine gas from unvented swimming pool areas; fungi growing in indoor plants and on the walls and floors of wet buildings; house mites in dirty carpets; dander from cats and dogs; toxic fumes from printed materials, copiers, and cleaning solutions (See Chapter Notes). The risk increases for a person who follows a low fat, low calorie diet, smokes, has weak lungs, or is elderly.

Let Them Eat Fat

The more malnourished you become, the more your respiratory disease will increase. Therefore, adequate nutrition and exercise cannot be underestimated in rebuilding respiratory muscles and improving energy. I recommend the "Pulmonary Diet" for anyone who is conscious of the need for increased breathing (dypsnea). This diet puts less stress on the lungs, it is divided into six meals and consists of 43 percent of the calories in fat and 43 percent in carbohydrates.[26] Dr. Jeffrey Askanzi nixes high carbohydrate diets for patients at risk for pulmonary breakdown and suggests adding only 300 calories over the amount their body needs. I base the caloric content on the person's lean tissue weight. Too many calories can overload the other systems, according to Dr. Askanzi. However, the very act of eating may exhaust people, so I suggest people try a formula, Pulmocare, which has been specially designed for people with Chronic Obstructive Pulmonary Disease (COPD). Actually, the formula can be consumed by anyone who needs a high fat diet. It can be ordered from a pharmacist. People who drink this formula need to drink a glass of water with it to prevent diarrhea (See Appendix for "Pulmonary Diet").

Adding isometric exercises can strengthen respiratory muscles. However, before trying exercise, people with lung diseases should receive permission from their physician and have a pulmonary function test. After exercising for two weeks, people had an overall feeling of well being.

If a person has lung and intestinal tract problems, I suggest they combine the Safe Diet with the Pulmonary Diet.

Eric had been unable to play outdoors for years. He had asthma. He developed skills in art and was a wonderful artist at the age of eight. Wistfully he watched the other children playing outdoors. But if he went out, he would wheeze and could not get his breath. This scared him. He was not allowed to run. He took all kinds of medication—antibiotics, puffers, inhalers, and antihistamine syrup. I designed a meal plan for him that had 45 percent fat, 12 percent protein and 43 percent carbohydrate. He needed the nutrients from complex carbohydrates, so I asked his mother to eliminate sweets and caffeine. After following the meal plan for three weeks, he ventured outside to play. He did not wheeze. He gained three pounds of lean tissue during the first six weeks that I worked with him.

The Pulmonary Diet is not well known nor publicized in this world of low fat and fat free diet hysteria. However, for anyone with breathing problems, it is worth a trial and worth continuing if it makes you feel better. The only warning I have is this. Don't go overboard and consume more fat or calories than is recommended.

Take time to smell the roses, taste and enjoy your food, be active and energetic and breathe in the wonderful air on a clear day! Happy Breathing!

Chapter Notes:

1: The pair of lungs in our body are beautifully designed with 750 million little balloon like air sacs that inflate when the oxygen enters and deflate when carbon dioxide is excreted. It is very rhythmic. In and out, in and out 14 to 18 times a minute. The lung never goes on vacation. As air is inhaled, it enters through the mouth and nose, travels down the trachea through the bronchial tubes, and into the air sacs. The air sacs release the oxygen into tiny blood vessels. The hemoglobin in the red blood cells picks up the oxygen and the blood distributes it to every cell. In the cell, the oxygen combusts with glucose or fat to create energy. One of the waste products from this combustion is carbon dioxide. It is carried back through the veins to the air sacs in the lungs and expelled from the body. The air sacs contain a protein called elastin that allows the balloon like sacs to inflate and deflate. The ribs of the lungs are connected by the muscles to the ribs with connective tissue and the connective tissue allows the lungs to breathe. The enzymes and counter enzymes in the lungs protect the body cells from inhaled smoke, bacteria, and pollutants.

2: Protease is the enzyme produced in the lungs which digests pollutants into harmless particles. However, it is also capable of digesting the protein in any cell. To prevent the protein in elastin and connective tissue from being digested by the protease, a hormone called alpha 1 anti-trysin (ATT) is also produced by the lung. But it too contains some protein which can be recruited for glucose. Without a counter balance ATT, the protease has free rein to digest the elastin and connective tissue. If the protein in the protease is recruited for glucose, then the inhaled pollutants are left to damage the air sacs and blood vessels.

3: One in 100 smokers have the ATT, a genetic defect. They develop emphysema at a very early age. Other smokers become malnourished or their lungs produce too much of the protease enzyme which eats not only bacteria and pollutants but bits of elastin and connective tissue cells as well, and they develop emphysema later. Smokers are six times more likely to die of emphysema or chronic bronchitis as non-smokers. Sixty five percent of smokers eventually develop emphysema. Others may develop cancer. Fatalities among American smokers each year from emphysema are 60,000 and from heart disease, 115,000.

4: Each year, 160,000 Americans die of carcinoma from smoking. Carcinoma arises in the cells of the body such as the skin, lips, surface of the cervix, linings of the mouth, larynx, trachea, bronchial tubes, esophagus, stomach, and rectum.

5: The cilia are hair projectiles that grow in the mucous of the nose, throat, and lungs. They sweep back and forth cleaning out toxins, germs, mucous, and dirt before they enter the lungs. When the nerve endings are destroyed, the lungs become the depository. For instance, the tar in nicotine, settles into the spongy cells of the body's air filtering system. Symptom: a persistent cough.

6: Smoking depletes vitamin C in the body resulting in a lower immune system, gum lesions, rough and scaly skin, soft and painful bones and even depression. With vitamin C's depletion, the immune system is impaired, increasing the vulnerability to cancer of the lungs, throat, and other organs. Without vitamin C in the meals, blood vessels can hemorrhage, muscles can degenerate and wounds can fail to heal. Vitamin C is found in fresh fruits and vegetables.

7: Other pollutants are carbon dioxide emitted by many people crammed into a small unventilated room; carbon monoxide from unvented garages; algae growing in fish tanks and dehumidifiers; virus and bacteria from room air conditioners; benzene and toluene from solvents and gasoline fumes.

8: To improve the strength of the respiratory muscles, people should start aerobic and anaerobic isometric exercises slowly and gradually increase the pace. Research reports a definite increase in quadricep and hamstring strength and leg muscle endurance after only two weeks of a isometric exercises. The report noted that the only limitation on exercise was shortness of breath, not leg muscle fatigue.

CHAPTER 9

Osteoporosis
Running Out Of Bone

A S unusual as it seems, bone does more than hold our body upright It is a pantry of nutrients and evergy which the body cells can snack on between meals. In fact, this critical function, many scientists believe, is one of bone's most important.

Usually bone is thought of as a solid foundation which never changes, similar to a cement foundation under a house. Unlike house foundations, bone is very much alive and responds to the demands of other cells. Bone can be torn down when the body cells tap its storage of nutrients. It rebuilds when the body receives enough nutrients and energy from food and the bone has stimulation from the muscles and hormones. So how in the world were calcium and estrogen singled out as the two substances that keep bones strong?

Perhaps calcium became the focus because it is a pivotal nutrient. No cell in the body can work unless it has calcium. That is why the body stores 99 percent in bone so it doesn't need to depend on the whim of what and when a person eats. But it is the other one percent that keeps us alive. Without calcium, the muscles cannot function, the heart cannot beat, nor the blood vessels contract and constrict. Blood cannot coagulate leading to hemorrhages and death from just a small cut. Nerve cells cannot carry messages from the brain.

The cells receive their calcium via the blood. Food supplies the calcium, and if it doesn't, it will be leached from bone, resulting in bone loss. If this continues over time, the bones can disintegrate into osteoporosis (See Chapter Notes for the definition of osteoporosis). When they do, they cease to be a reliable resource for the other body cells. Osteoporosis is a serious condition. When it develops in the early years, the bone becomes soft and bend resulting in bowed legs. When it develops in the older years, it becomes hollow and can no longer hold you erect (See Chapter Notes). The health of the bones reflects your health from childhood. Taking measures in your younger years can prevent osteoporosis from developing in your older years.

To the unwary and nutritionally unsophisticated, ingesting a calcium supplement may seem to be the solution to prevent osteoporosis. How simple and easy that would be. However, much of the credit given to calcium belongs to the other players, other nutrients, calories, exercise, and hormones. There is a whole fascinating game of nutrition dominos being played between the body cells and the bone cells with the blood carrying the nutrients back and forth.

Two hormones, not supplements or food, control the amount of calcium carried in the blood (See Chapter Notes). The hormones stimulate bone to pick up calcium or release it as the calcium levels in the blood rise or fall. The two hormones maintain a ratio of two parts calcium to one part phosphorus.

The amount of calcium which can enter the blood from food depends heavily on a healthy intestinal tract and healthy kidneys.

Bone cells increase when muscles pull on them whether from exercise or from added body weight. The opposite is also true. When a person does not exercise at least three days a week or loses weight, the number of bone cells can dwindle. They dwindle if meals are skipped, eating becomes erratic, dieting continuously to lose weight or consuming too few calories to support your lean tissue (See Chapter Notes).

Bones contain protein like any other cell in the body. The protein forms a woven fabric upon which glucose deposits the minerals, calcium, phosphorus, magnesium, and fluoride (See Chapter Notes) and creates an armor-like structure. Without protein, the base is gone and so are the contents of the bone cell.

The marrow of the bone contains ferritin, another protein. Ferritin, combined with iron, produces hemoglobin. The liver can recruit ferritin for glucose and when it does, you become anemic. Anemia is a condition which occurs also when something traumatic occurs to the bone like a break or surgery. Anemia can also be an early indicator of osteoporosis.

Enemies of Bone

Substances that interfere with bone building are diuretics, laxatives, and medications.

Diuretics stimulate the kidney to excrete sodium and water from the blood (water makes up 93 percent of the plasma of the blood). When water leaves, so do the water soluble bone building materials such as minerals, vitamins, and amino acids. It seems fruitless to take a calcium and/or a magnesium supplement to replace these nutrients when diuretics flush them from the body too quickly for the bone to absorb them.

Alcoholic and caffeinated beverages and some medications act as diuretics. Research[23] shows that diveretics cause less calcium loss and reduces estrogen production in post menopausal women increasing their risk of Osteoporotic fractures (See Appendix for sources of Caffeine). Soft drinks deliver a double whammy to bones with their phosphoric acid content and the caffeine.

Betty was 70 years of age. She had many physical complaints, including high blood pressure. I measured her height and wrist and I provided her with a meal plan to support her lean tissue. I also suggested that she eliminate the soft drinks and coffee, reduce her meat intake from six to eight ounces to two ounces at a meal and exercise aerobically 30 minutes a day. A few months later her blood pressure dropped to normal and her physician told her she could eliminate the diuretic medication. A year later, I measured her wrist and her height. Both of us were amazed. Her wrist had grown one quarter of an inch and her height, one half inch.

Alcohol can create more problems than caffeine, especially for those Americans who have two drinks daily. The alcohol destroys bones gradually, like water eroding cement. Alcohol stimulates the parathyroid hormone to release calcium from bone. It prevents the kidney from recycling bone building nutrients. It stops the kidney from converting vitamin D to calcitriol, a hormone necessary to stimulate the intestinal tract to absorb calcium. It can damage the cells in the intestinal tract, interfering with the digestion of calcium. The process of storing vitamin A in the liver can be hindered, and the production of glucose, the bones' source of energy, can be inhibited.

Alcohol can suppress a person's appetite, thereby denying the body its source of vitamin A and other bone building materials. The net result from alcohol consumption over time is osteoporosis, osteomalacia, bowed legs, and therefore, weak knees.

Medications can affect the level of blood calcium by interfering with the absorption of bone building nutrients.

Tobacco use not only indirectly destroys bones by robbing the body of calcium, but it inhibits the absorption of vitamin D and magnesium. It is also interferes with oxygen intake. Oxygen is necessary to create energy so that the hormones, the intestinal tract, and the kidneys can work to directly or indirectly supply calcium for the blood.

Illnesses, an unhealthy intestinal tract, or unhealthy kidneys automatically predispose a person to osteoporosis. For instance, with diarrhea, the nutrients pass through the intestinal tract too fast to be absorbed. Laxatives create the same problem.

Calcium: How Much is Too Much

Dietary sources of bone building nutrients are always preferable. Calcium is only one bone building nutrient and cannot replace the macro-nutrients or other bone building nutrients (See Chapter Notes for sources of calcium). However, in a few instances a calcium supplement may be necessary. When calcium supplements are used, they should be considered just that: supplement to the calcium obtained from dietary sources. Since the bone cells of an adult normally pick up about 300 to 400 mg of calcium at any one time, the total mix between the meal and the supplement should approximate that amount. Ingesting calcium in these small amounts increases the absorption rate and does not increase the alkalin of the stomach, intestinal tract, or urinary tract.

If more calcium is ingested, the kidneys must excrete the excess or the calcium builds up as calcium stones and/or it is deposited in such soft tissue as the lungs and breasts. A person will know if they are taking too much. It will make them feel dizzy, weak and lethargic. Also, calcium, as in antacids, taken in large doses can reduce the acidity of the stomach. It is important that the stomach be somewhat acidic otherwise it reduces the ability of the intestinal tract to absorb calcium, zinc, magnesium, and iron. Additionally, if it is found necessary to drink cranberry juice to keep the urinary tract more alkaline, it makes more sense to first eliminate the possible causes such as antacids and calcium supplements.

Everytime a person exercises, magnesium trades places with calcium. It leaves the bone and enters the blood where it make itself available to the muscles, such as the heart and lungs (See Chapter Notes for sources of magnesium).

The Pros and Cons of Estrogen

With interactions between nutrients and hormones so complex and interdependent, how did estrogen acquire such a glamorous image? Perhaps estrogen became the target because so many more women than men develop osteoporosis. Perhaps it was because research found that 300 different tissues respond to estrogen. Some of these tissues are the bones, brain, skin, breasts, urinary tract, genitalia, and liver (See Chapter Notes).

And as women approach menopause, their ovaries produce less estrogen with changes appearing in the tissues that need it. Their skin becomes drier, their hair becomes gray and more brittle, the hair under their arms and between the legs becomes sparse, their urinary tract and genitalia become more dry, moods change, and metabolism slows.

However, estrogen does not act alone any more than calcium acts alone. In fact, if it weren't for the other hormones, (hypothalamus, pituitary, and thyroid) there would be no estrogen. The pituitary stimulates the ovaries where estrogen is produced and, in turn, the hypothalamus stimulates the pituitary. The pituitary controls so many other hormones, that it is called the master gland. It also balances the fluid in the body. The hypothalamus affects other hormones, but it especially controls metabolism and the body thermostat.

As one ages, the hormones act like a house of cards. When one hormone slows down they all slow down. Women who have the greatest risk for sluggish hormones are thin and Caucasian, with very little body fat. Body fat produces a form of estrogen, estone. It would appear, then, that heavy women with more body fat have less of a risk for osteoporosis and less of a need for Estrogen Replacement Therapy (ERT).

For thin Caucasian women, ERT may slow the onset of osteoporosis for three to eight years after menopause, reduce hot flashes, irritable moods, and dry vaginas. Sometimes estrogen, in the form of birth control, is prescribed for young women to relieve cramping, irregular periods, or to produce menstrual periods. Perhaps their body fat is so low that their the hormones cannot stimulate the ovaries to produce enough estrogen and therefore they stop menstruating. When body fat is too low in men, their body produces less testosterone. Research[24] has found that less testosterone is a risk factor for bone deterioration. Women too produce some testosterone, but the amount depends on the estrogen hormone. Research[24] has also found that when the ovaries are removed surgically, testosterone production is reduced by one-third[25] It is thought that young women who do not produce enough estrogen or young men who do not produce enough testosterone, overexercise or undereat. Research reports that osteoporosis has been found in ballet dancers, runners who run more than 65 miles a week, and athletes who compete without eating enough calories.[26]

Amenorrhea (lack of menstruation) is not an exclusive problem with women who have low body fat. Cessation of menstruation can occur in overweight women too. Research[27] reports that women who did not menstruate regularly, ate erratically, skipped meals, were continuously dieting, and failed to eat enough calories and nutrients.

A woman age 22 with medium build, a little overweight, came to see me for a diet. Her nutrition history revealed that she ate what she wanted when she wanted it. She did not cook at home, so most of her food came from fast food restaurants or the vending machines. She had a low self esteem, had dropped out of high school and believed if she lost weight she would be more attractive. I provided her with a meal plan which supported her lean tissue weight. She followed the meal plan faithfully. Six weeks later she bounced in and announced, "I'm menstruating." She told me she had not menstruated since she was 12 years of age even though doctors had prescribed birth control pills. She believed something was wrong with her because she was not like the other girls. This condition contributed to her view of herself as an incomplete, unworthy female.

Food habits have more of a bearing on the onset of osteoporosis than estrogen ever can, in spite of ingesting the hormone. In no stretch of the imagination can estrogen replace regular meals which contain enough calories and nutrients to support lean tissue. Hormones which balance with estrogen need energy as much as any other part of the body.

ERT is prescribed for post menopausal women to revert or reduce the risk of osteoporosis. Can ERT be considered a miracle pill? Inherent in the presupposition that estrogen alone will slow the onset of osteoporosis is an underlying message. The message is that it doesn't matter what kind of lifestyle a woman had or continues to have, estrogen alone is the answer. The underlying message seems to say, it doesn't matter how much a women eats drinks, smokes, takes medications, or ingests vitamin and mineral supplements as long as they use the estrogen supplement. A similar message is being promoted by manufacturers who claim that estrogen will slow the onset of Alzheimer's and heart disease.

ERT does increase the total skeleton one to two percent but is that not enough to prevent fractures or increase bone mass? Osteoporosis aside, the safety of taking estrogen has not been answered yet. A study by the National Institutes of Health[28] will not be completed until 2003. In this study more than 140,000 volunteers are being given either a hormone or placebo over a period of years. Other studies have been completed. Long term[29] studies associated with using birth control medication report an increased risk for breast cancer, endometrial and pancreatic cancer, high blood pressure, strokes, heart disease, increased triglycerides, and sodium retention (See Chapter Notes about the side effect of estrogen). Between 1973 and 1988 the increase in breast cancer approached 26 percent. The conclusion by the Center for Disease Control: women using estrogen (birth control or ERT) for more than 15 years have a 30 percent increased risk for breast cancer.[30] Another study[31] reports that women using estrogen supplements for more than six years incur a 40 percent increased risk for ovarian cancer and, if taken for 11 years, incur a 70 percent risk. Combine smoking with ERT and the risk of cancer increases more than with estrogen alone. Women are faced with a choice between two risks—cancer and osteoporosis.

Another problem with ERT and birth control pills is the side effect of weight gain. On the positive side, bones respond to an increase in weight and become larger. Pregnant women can relate to this. As they gain weight, many have reported an increase in shoe size. Some of it may stem from the extra estrogen in their body, but more than likely, it is the additional weight. People who are heavier in their fifties may discover that they need a shoe size larger than what they wore in their twenties.

On the negative side, most women dislike gaining weight. Many women have told me they gained several pounds after starting ERT or birth control pills even though they had not changed their usual eating and drinking habits. This insidious side effect may not begin immediately, maybe not for years, but when it does, many women believe the weight gain is from eating too much. The women feel guilty. Their self esteem drops. They do not like the way they look, so they diet. They eat less fat but do not lose weight.

If the estrogen affects the intestinal tract and causes bloating, less bone building materials are absorbed, canceling out the benefits of the ERT.

Lizabeth had a hysterectomy at the age of 62. Following the operation, her physician prescribed large amounts of estrogen along with 1500 mg of calcium. She gained weight and dieted. When she was 72, she arose from a chair and her hip bone collapsed. She fell. She had a hip replacement and her diagnosis was osteoporosis. She could not walk without a great deal of pain in her back, so she also received pain medication. She developed high blood pressure and received diuretics and heart medication. She had no energy and did not feel well. Thinking she needed vitamins, she ingested large quantities. While she did not use tobacco or drink alcohol, she ate chocolate and drank coffee. She reduced her caloric intake to only 700 to 800 calories a day. Between the ages of 75 to 78 she fell many times and suffered several spinal vertebrae fractures even though she was still ingesting estrogen and large amounts of calcium. She had to resort to a wheelchair and eventually to a bed.

Controlling osteoporosis and cancer through nutrition and lifestyle choices does not raise questions about adverse reactions as it does from using estrogen or, for that matter, any medication used over the long term (See Chapter Notes about informed choices).

If women choose not to use estrogen, what can they do about hot flashes and dry vaginas? There are simple suggestions which are not broadcast by pharmaceutical manufacturers. For the hot flashes, women can try eliminating alcohol, nicotine, caffeine, and sugar and can consume adequate calories and nutrients to build up their lean tissue. For a dry vagina, which means dry mucous membranes, women can use over-the- counter water soluble lubricants and add more fat to their low fat diet. Adding more dietary fat attracts more vitamin A. Vitamin A is needed to thicken the mucous membranes.

Males *Versus* Females

Men can develop osteoporosis too. It develops more slowly. After the age 70, men catch up with women and have almost as many hip and vertebral fractures.

Males in their teen years usually build more bone than women because men are usually not as diet conscious, eat more food, are generally more active physically, and have more lean tissue weight. They also do not bear children. Since men start out with more bone, their risk for developing osteoporosis early in life is not as great However, there is a pocket of men, about *five* percent, under the age of 70 who are at risk. Their risk factors are overexercising, low body fat, low testosterone levels, illness, and emphysema.

As both men and women age, the balance of hormones changes, the stomach produces less acid, the ability of the kidneys to convert vitamin D to calcitriol is reduced, the cells work less efficiently, less nutrients are absorbed regardless of supplement strength, and more nutrients are released at a faster rate from bone. All men and women after age 70 obviously experience some osteoporosis. But theirs is not a result of estrogen or testosterone loss. Rather, it is related to aging of all cells, cells which are compromised by numerous factors. The most important of which is food.

CHAPTER 9a

Early Warning Signs

YOU may think that osteoporosis is an old person's disease. Yes, old age is when osteoporosis is most visible and when people suffer the most from it. Osteoporosis, however, does not begin in old age. The deterioration of the bones begins much earlier. In fact, the health of the bones is a reflection of your lifestyle, physical activity, and nutritional history (See Chapter Notes to evaluate the risk for developing osteoporosis). Bones can be healthy and their deterioration can be delayed if you know the early warning signs and take action.

Signs of Shrinking Bone

- A toothbrush that has pink bristles after teeth are brushed
- Fast weight loss in a short period of time
- Loss of height
- Back pain
- Bowed legs
- Slow mending of broken bones

Unhealthy Teeth

Teeth are a window into the health of the rest of the body. Barring a genetic weakness, teeth deteriorate because the body is sick or is malnourished or they aren't maintained regularly with brushing, flossing, and professional cleanings. Teeth deteriorate because the gums break down. The gums bleed preventing the teeth from being nourished. Eventually, the teeth can fall out, resulting in chewing problems and further malnourishment.

Fast Weight Loss

Bones respond to weight changes in both men and women. When a person loses a great deal of weight, they place their body at risk for many medical problems, one of which is early osteoporosis. Excessive weight loss may be the result of inadequate nutrition and food withheld over a period of time.

Women who are overweight and want to lose weight, often tell me they want to weigh what they did in high school. When I measure them, their lean tissue weight is often greater than what they remember as their total weight in high school. Part of the increase in their lean tissue weight is bone cells. I use the following as an explanation. I compare their skeleton to a coat rack. The skeleton is that on which their flesh hangs. With the coat rack, the more coats on the coat rack, the larger the rack must be. The more flesh added to the skeleton, the larger the skeleton must grow to hold it up. People probably may not realize that bones cells are alive and can grow or deteriorate even in the adult years.

When Mary Jean was 20 years old she weighed 120 pounds with a possible lean tissue weight of 100 pounds. She gained weight over the next 20 years to 280 pounds, and her lean tissue weight was 168 pounds. An obvious sign was the size of her wrists. They were extremely large.

Loss of Height

As people approach middle age, they may become shorter. Changes in bone loss can be detected by measuring height or arm span yearly. Arm span that exceeds height indicates vertebrae loss. Following menopause, a woman can shrink as much as 1.5 inches in height over a period of ten years. The key here is "as much as." In other words it is not a definite prediction.

Back Pain

A backache can signal the deterioration of the vertebrae (spinal column bones) and is one of the early signs of osteoporosis. Another way to detect early bone deterioration is a bone density or blood test (See Chapter Notes). The deterioration of the vertebrae means they are becoming hollow and the weight of the body mass can crush the hollow bones. Each crush fracture causes a reduction in the height by 1 centimeter. If the bone density or blood test determines that you have osteoporosis and do not change your lifestyle and nutrition habits, the vertebrae will continue to shrink. Your body contour will change. A stoop will become obvious as the shoulders, neck and head thrust forward, the waistline enlarges and the stomach pouches out. The organs become crowded, forcing changes in the intestine, stomach, lungs and kidneys.

Bowed Legs

As unusual as it may seem, most men do not develop bowed legs from riding horses. Instead their bowed legs are more than likely the result of overconsumption of protein and/or phosphorus. Perhaps they eat two or three hamburgers at a sitting, 12 to 24 ounce steaks at meals, ingest amino acid supplements or protein rich formulas in an attempt to enlarge their muscles. Women can develop bowed legs by frequently consuming liquid protein formulas or meat and salad regimes in their attempt to lose weight. The bowed legs can be a result of consuming several soft drinks on a daily basis. If this is the way you feed your body, you are not only loading up with protein and amino acids, but your diet is lacking many other nutrients including bone building nutrients. All it takes to lose one to one and one half percent of the skeletal mass annually, is a 50 percent increase consumption of dietary protein.[32] A 50 percent increase of protein is only three ounces of meat when you compare it to the recommended allotment of two ounces. Men who consume 12 ounce steaks are consuming a 600 percent increase in protein.

While the protein and the soft drinks contain phosphorus, so do a lot of other foods (See Chapter Notes for sources of phosphorus). In the last 20 years the amount of phosphorus added to food has increased 200 percent and to soft drinks, 300 percent. As long ago as 1974, scientist Leo Lutwak[33] sounded a warning that the ratio of phosphorus consumption in America at that time was one part calcium to four parts phosphorus, a striking imbalance when the hormones are programmed to maintain it at two parts calcium to one part phosphorus. When milk is regularly replaced with soft drinks, and the foods containing calcium are replaced with fast and convenience foods containing large amounts of phosphorus additives, at least two negatives can result. The bones can be drained of calcium, making them weaker, softer, and curved, and the kidney undergoes stress to excrete many times more phosphorus than it did 20 years ago. Bones depleted of calcium not only curve but can break. Research[34] reports that there is a 2.28 greater incidence of fractures in athletes over the age of 40 who drink carbonated beverages compared to athletes who drink water.

Bones Slow to Mend

The time it takes for broken bones to mend depends on the condition of your body before and how well you feed it after the break. The trauma of a broken bone or a bone which is surgically repaired affects the whole body—a body which can lose weight, become anemic, weaker, and less resistant to infections. The lost weight and anemia are signs of lost lean tissue weight, some of which is bone cells. Repairing bones and other vital parts requires more calories and nutrients than does maintenance. Yet how many people are reminded to eat more when they break a bone?

Filling Up Your Local Bone Tank for the Long Haul

Building bone is complicated and is not a one nutrient or one hormone issue. Nutritionally, to build or repair bone, nutrients must come from all six food groups with enough calories to support lean tissue (2000 calories for women, 2400 for men or more per day) (See Meal Plans in appendix). The Milk Group provides a large mix of bone building materials.

To give a synopsis of how nutrients from food build your bone let's take one meal. You choose to eat some starches which will provide energy (glucose) and nutrients. You choose something from the Milk Group and the calcium enters the stomach with some fruit you have chosen. The vitamin C in the fruit adds some acid to the stomach. In this acidic environment, the calcium and other nutrients are changed into a soluble form of single molecules that the intestinal tract can absorb. You choose some butter from the Fat Group which helps absorb the vitamin D from Milk, the vitamin A from butter and from vegetables. You chose a food from the Meat Group, which supplies zinc, the mineral which stimulates the liver to release its storage of vitamin A. The vitamin A keeps the absorptive mucous membranes healthy and prepares old bone materials for new. Hormones in the kidneys stimulate the cells in the intestinal tract to absorb the calcium and other bone building materials which enter the blood stream. The calcitonin and parathyroid hormones do a dance so to speak and, as the blood calcium moves toward the bone, the phosphorus from the Meat Group and milk from the Milk Group help the bones absorb it.

Of course, more nutrients will be absorbed by the bone if you exercise. The muscle will pull on the bone and stimulate it.

More nutrients will be absorbed if you place limits on protein, nicotine, and some other medications. The misuse of these substances can be a greater contributing factor than inadequate calcium or estrogen to the development of osteoporosis.

Bone is a pantry of nutrients which the rest of the body can tap. The magical image that has been given to calcium and estrogen may have brought attention to the public about the seriousness of osteoporosis, but preventing osteoporosis is much more complicated than just ingesting two substances.

The safest course you can take to prevent the body from robbing the bone of its nutrients is to have an 80 year plan. Plan to keep your bones filled every day with enough nutrients and energy to support your lean tissue. Plan to exercise. Plan to eliminate offending substances. Plan to take the time to "smell the roses," and plan to sleep eight solid hours each day.

You have a choice: letting your bones be robbed of their nutrients so that they shrink and curve, or having a straight back at age 80 and enjoying life almost as much as you did in your youth.

Chapter Notes:

1: Osteoporosis is derived from the Greek words "osteo" meaning bone, from "poros" meaning porous, and from "osis" meaning condition. Osteoporosis means limited freedom and is a serious condition. The number of fractures caused by osteoporosis (one million) in 1993 was greater than the number of heart attacks and strokes (741,000) or the number of cancer cases (257,000). Over 40,000 American women die from its complications each year.

2: The bones are encased in a hard shell. The compact bone surrounding the shaft of the long bones such as arms and leg, hands and feet is the cortical bone. Beneath the shell are crisscrossed bony fibers of the trabeculae. Inside the bone is the soft fatty material of the marrow where ferritin is stored and joins with iron to make red blood cells. Trabecular bone takes up 20 percent of the body skeleton. Yet it is trabecular bone that gives up the calcium to replenish blood calcium. And as it does, the inside of the bone becomes hollow. The first bones to give way are the vertebrae, then the ribs, and lastly the long bones. As the vertebrae become weak, they are crushed by the weight of the body mass. The spine reaches a point where it can no longer hold the body erect, reducing the quality of life.

3: Sources of Phosphorus: Meats, soft drinks, processed cheese, ice cream, additives such as stabilizers, baking powder (sodium aluminum phosphate), monocalcium phosphate, and sodium phosphate, aluminum phosphate, potassium phosphate, sodium tripolyphosphate, dipotassium phosphate, calcium phosphate, diammonium phosphate.

4: How calcium enters the blood from the intestinal tract. First, the calcium must go through an acid stomach to change it to a form that can be digested in the small intestine. The next move before calcium can enter the blood lies with the kidney. A healthy kidney converts vitamin D to the calcitriol hormone. Vitamin D is produced when the sun triggers a chemical reaction with cholesterol under the skin and then it is stored in the liver until the kidney needs it. The calcitriol hormone stimulates the intestinal tract to absorb calcium and other nutrients into the blood. As blood passes through the kidney, the kidney is stimulated by the calcitriol hormone to return 400 mg of calcium to the blood over a period of 24 hours. Exposing one's skin to the sun 15 to 20 minutes converts the cholesterol under the skin to vitamin D3. Statistics show that greater numbers of Caucasians suffer from osteoporosis than those of the darker skinned races because dark skin absorbs more rays from the sun than light skin. Vitamin D3 is also found in cod liver oil, egg yolk, saltwater fish, and liver. A synthetic vitamin D developed in the 1940's was added to foods, especially to milk. However, it is not added to cottage cheese, yogurt, ice cream, or goat's milk.

5: Bones are made up of cells. The more cells in the bone, the more dense and strong it is, and the better it is able to hold up the tissue that clings to it. The 206 bones in the skeleton protect the delicate organs and tissues within. They are like tubes with an outer hard shell and an inner core. The outer shell and inner core are made up of billions, maybe trillions of cells. Nutrients fill the cells, providing density. These stored nutrients are what the body cells depend on when invaded by infections or disease. But in giving up these nutrients, the bone cells silently die. As more and more bone cells die in the early years, they become soft and curved. Gums bleed and women stop menstruating. In the later years, deterioration of bone means the loss of cells from the inner core. They become hollow while the outer shell becomes pitted and porous, brittle and dried out. The bone becomes vulnerable to cracks and fractures. Such bone is similar to a clam shell that has been eroded by sea water.

6: Conditions which reduce the body's ability to absorb calcium are caloric restriction, illness or a disease, stress, and regular use of some medications (See Chapter Notes).

7: When a person consumes inadequate calories, the blood becomes more acidic. To restore the acid base balance, bone releases sodium. It keeps 30 to 45 percent of the body's total amount of sodium on its surface so that it is readily available whenever the blood becomes even slightly acidic. When sodium leaves though, large amounts of calcium are drained from the bones. The consequence is a loss of lean tissue cells, including those in bone.

8: There are many medications and drugs which can prevent the absorption of bone building materials. They include: Cholestryamine (Questran and Cholybar) which are prescribed to control blood cholesterol.

Glucocorticosteroids such as Prednisone and Corticol convert vitamin D to an inactive form. Therefore calcium cannot be absorbed.

Diuretics force the excretion of bone building nutrients along with sodium and water. Hydrochlorothiazide (HCTZ) prevents calcium excretion but leads to the excretion of other bone building nutrients.

Phenobarbital, an anticonvulsant medication accelerates the use of vitamin D resulting in large amounts of calcium and magnesium being excreted. Dilantin prevents the absorption of vitamin D3 contributing to rickets in children and osteoporosis in adults.

Bisacodyl, (Ducolax), a laxative, can mean the loss of potassium and, if taken with milk, will bind up calcium. Two other laxatives, mineral oil and caster oil, coat the lining of the intestinal tract preventing nutrients from being absorbed. Other laxatives can depress appetite. A drug which prevents the absorption of bone building materials is nicotine which inhibits the absorption of vitamin D3 and magnesium and indirectly destroys bone by robbing the body of calcium.

9: Dietary sources of Calcium:

Dairy products are the source of 75 percent of calcium and this source has a greater absorption rate than others.

Yogurt—skim and low fat	8 oz	415
Fruit yogurt	8 oz	343
Sardines—packed in oil	3 oz	372
Skim Milk	8 oz	302
Low fat Milk—1%	8 oz	300
Low fat Milk—2%	8 oz	297
Whole milk—4%	8 oz	291
Buttermilk—cultured	8 oz	285
Chocolate Milk—2%	8 oz	284
Chocolate Milk—whole	8 oz	280
Ricotta Cheese—part skim	4 oz	335
Mozzarella Cheese—part skim	1 oz	207

Other sources of calcium that are well absorbed are:

Oysters, canned salmon, goat's milk, cornmeal tortillas soaked in calcium rich lime, soybeans (tofu), chicken and pork broth made with bones boiled in vinegar, orange juice and flour with added calcium. Hard water with lime contains calcium.

There is calcium in the following but it is bound up in oxalic salt and phytic acid and the body does not have the ability to break the calcium out and thus, to absorb it: spinach, kale, broccoli, mustard greens, collards and turnip greens. If oxalates as in rhubarb, chocolate, chard and beet greens are at the same time as foods which contain calcium, the oxalates interfere with calcium's absorption.

10: Each time the heart beats or the lungs inhale or exhale, calcium does a little dance of sorts with magnesium. A little magnesium exits the bone and enters the muscles and a little calcium enters bone. This too lends credence to the idea that bone acts more as a supply depot for other body cells than as a structural support (As much as 60 percent of the bodies' total supply of magnesium is stored in bone). The more a person exercises, the greater the exchange and the stronger the bones become, as long as the person eats the fruits and vegetables along with foods from other groups.

11: As a child grows, so do the hormones. Estrogen production rises gradually in childhood and gradually recedes before and after menopause. As less estrogen is being produced, the hypothalamus revs up and keeps stimulating the ovaries to produce estrogen. The estrogen level rises and falls erratically. Menstruation becomes less regular and usually stops after five years. In the meantime, the overactive hypothalamus triggers hot flashes, a faster heartbeat, and nighttime sweats.

12: The side effects of estrogen either taken as birth control pills or as ERT are weight gain, headaches, cancer of the uterus, breast and other organs, endometriosis, abnormal vaginal bleeding, vaginal yeast infections, depression, arthritis, swelling of the breasts thrombosis, increased blood cholesterol and triglycerides. Others are sudden dizziness, difficulty in speaking, numbness or tingling in the body, constipation, feeling faint, sudden shortness of breath, yellowing of the eyes and skin, dark-colored urine, itching, sudden changes in vision, flashes of light before the eyes, and focusing difficulties.

13: Making informed choices:

Women with a hereditary predisposition to cancer generally are not candidates for ERT. Cancer isn't caused by estrogen, but estrogen can accelerate its growth if the cancer cells are present.

Women who have fibroid tumors, endometriosis, blood clotting or bleeding problems are not candidates for ERT. Neither are women who have liver or gall bladder diseases.

Women with high blood pressure, diabetes, heart disease, or who ingest vitamin C in large doses (1000 mg or more per day), or who use medications such as Prednisone, or anti-inflammatory drugs are not candidates for ERT.

14: You can delay osteoporosis. To evaluate your risk, you can take an inventory based on the following questions. This modified questionnaire is based on a point system developed by Dr. Kenneth Cooper, an internationally known author and physician. It is also based on the research which is used in this chapter.

The point system is not exact but can give you an idea of your risks. The more questions to which you answer yes, the greater your risk. Low risk is 0-10 points. Moderate risk is 11-20 points, high risk is 21-30. Above 31 the risk is very great.

Risk Factor	No. of Points	YES	NO
Are you a woman?	3		
Are you over 50 years of age?	3		
Did your parents have osteoporosis?	2		
Are you Caucasian and have fair complexion?	2		
Do you exercise aerobically less than 30 minutes three times a week?	3		
Have you been bedridden over time?	10		
Is your body fat less than 15 percent?	4		
Are you dieting, have anorexia nervosa or bulimia?	4		
Do you consume less than 2000 calories/day?	4		
Do you *eat* less than three meals daily?	4		
Do you eat less than 15 grams of fat/meal?	2		
For how many meals do you eat less than a half serving from the Milk Group?Less than three?	3		
For how many meals do you eat more than 3 oz from the Meat Group? More than three?	3		
Are you a vegetarian who does not eat servings from the Meat or Milk Group?	3		
Do you drink alcoholic beverages? More than 2 ounces of alcohol a day?	4		
Do you drink caffeinated beverages? More than four a day?	3		
Less than two a day?	2		
Do you smoke?	4		
Do you have intestinal problems?	3		
Do you have diarrhea?	4		
Do you take the following medications: (See Chapter Notes)			

Laxatives?	3	
Tetracycline?	3	
Antibiotics?	3	
For high blood cholesterol?	3	
Diuretics?	3	
Antacids?	3	
Anticonvulsant or anti-glaucoma?	3	
Corticosteroids like Prednisone?	4	
Anti-inflammatory?	4	
Transplant?	4	
Do you sleep more than eight hours a day?	2	
Do you have any diseases such as diabetes, cancer, hormone deficiencies, kidney disease, or overactive thyroid?	15	
Do you take megadoses of vitamin and mineral supplements?	4	
Do you use street drugs such as marijuana cocaine, etc.?	4	
	Total	Total

15: Physicians can detect the onset of osteoporosis early by sophisticated measures which in the past were only detected later in life. One which many use is the Osteogram which is a computer analysis X-Ray of the hand. It determines the person's bone mineral density. The dose of the radiation is minimal and is comparable to a panoramic dental X-Ray.

CHAPTER 10

Sources Of Fuel And Raw Materials

The Four Step System

THERE is a system to ensure that your body receives the 60 nutrients in the quantities established for you by the Food and Nutrition Board of the National Academy of Sciences[36] (See Appendix D). The system has four steps. The first is determining the number of calories you need. The second is dividing them into three meals. The third is following the outline below and the final step is choosing the foods.

(See Chapter 2 to find out how you determine the number of calories you need).

The number of calories for each meal will be 600 to 750 calories if it is based on 2000 (for a woman) and 2400 (for a man) calories per day respectively.

When you choose foods as outlined here you will fulfill the recommended percentages of protein, carbohydrate and fat.

Each meal will have 12 to 15 percent in *protein*, 55-60 percent in *carbohydrate*, and 25 to 30 percent in *fat*.

For the amount of *protein* you need choose:

Two ounces from the *Meat Group* and one-half serving from the *Milk Group*.

For the amount of *carbohydrate* you need choose:

Three to five servings from the *Starch Group* (depending on your caloric needs) and one or two from the *Fruit Group*

For the *fat* you can choose:

One to three servings, depending on the amount of fat in the foods you chose from the *Meat and Milk Groups*.

The *fat* content should be 18 to 22 gms a meal.

For the *rest of the nutrients*, you can choose a serving from the *Vegetable Group* at each of two meals.

For the *snack:*

You can choose a serving from the *Milk or Meat Groups* to provide some *protein*. And add a serving from the *Starch* or *Fruit group* to provide some *carbohydrate*. Calories should total about 200.

To ensure you receive the nutrients in a timely manner you can feed your body a meal about every *five hours*.

Nutrients depends on each other's presence. They can work more efficiently if they can interact as they travel through the intestinal tract and liver. Therefore, with this in mind, the meals are designed to incorporate the 60 into each meal. If the nutrients are separated by hours, less of them are able to interact with each other. Take just two nutrients. *Iron* in foods from the *Meat Group* depends on *vitamin C* being present as it is absorbed in the intestinal tract. The orange juice at breakfast will no longer be in the stomach when the iron in the hamburger arrives at noon. Some nutrients in foods are stored and released during digestion and absorption, but the majority are not.

Many nutrients consumed in excess are not saved in the stomach or the intestinal tract or anywhere else to be available at the time they are needed during digestion and absorption. For instance, when a person eats an eight ounce steak, the amount of protein that the cells can extract and use is only the amount from about three ounces. Protein is not stored. The remainder is stored as fat (See Appendix for sample meal plans for 2000, 2200, 2400 calories, respectively).

Nutrients

The body cells need 60 nutrients. The amount of each nutrient, except for fat and carbohydrates, has been determined by the Food and Nutrition Board of the National Academy of Sciences for each age and sex. The only source for *all* 60 nutrients is food. The word "food" means it contains nutrients and calories in its natural state.

Foods can be classified according to their nutrients and gathered into Groups. The nutrients in each food group are unique to that group and not provided in sufficient quantities by any other food group. Some food groups overlap a few nutrients. There are six food groups: *Meat, Milk, Fat, Starch, Vegetables* and *Fruit*. When you eat a food from each food group in sufficient quantities you will have consumed the amounts of the nutrients recommended for you.

The Six Food Groups

Meat Group

Each ounce of meat or the equivalent (as listed below) has approximately 75 calories and about the same amount of protein, zinc, iron, copper, B 12, phosphorus. The white "meats" such as turkey, and fish have less iron and less fat but contain some vitamin B6 as does egg yolk.

Meat and poultry (beef, lamb, pork, liver, chicken, turkey, venison, etc.)
One egg
Fish:

Codfish, mackerel, orange roughy, etc.	1 slice (2" x 2")
Salmon, tuna, crab (fresh or 1/4 cup if canned in w water)	2 oz
Oysters, shrimp, clams	5 sm
Sardines—packed in water	3 med

Milk Group

The size portion of products listed below contain about the same amount of protein, calcium, riboflavin, phosphorus, and B 12. The difference in the calories is largely due to the fat content.

Whole Milk,	1 cup	160 Cal
Plain Yogurt,	1 cup	150 Cal
Milk, Evaporated,	1/2 cup	160 Cal
Cheeses, Cheddar, Colby		
Milk, powdered,	1/4 cup	90 Cal
	1 1/2 oz	170 Cal
Buttermilk, Cottage Cheese,		
Low Fat	1 cup	90 Cal
Milk, 2%,	1 cup	120 Cal
	1/2 cup	185 Cal
Milk, Skim & 1/2%,	1 cup	90 Cal
Cottage Cheese reg or 4%	1/2 cup	115 Cal

Starch Group

Each size portion below contains approximately 70 calories, complex carbohydrates, some of the Vitamin B's, and fiber, especially if it is whole grain or eaten with the skin.

Bread	1 slice
Bagel	1/2
Bun, Hamburger or hot dog	1/2
Biscuits, roll	1 or 2" diam
Muffin	1 or 2" diam
Cornbread	1 1/2" cube
Taco shell, tortilla	1
Cereal, dry, flaked	3/4 cup
Cereal, cooked	1/2 cup
Pasta, (noodles, spaghetti, macaroni)	1/2 cup
Crackers, graham	2
Crackers, saltine	5
Crackers, round	6
Pancake, 6" round	1

Vegetables:

Parsnips	2/3 cup
Beans, Dry, Cooked (Navy) Lima, Split Pea	1/2 cup
Baked Beans, no fat	1/4 cup
Corn	1/3 cup
Popcorn	3 cups
Potatoes, white, baked or no fat	1 (2" diam)
Potatoes, white, mashed, or boiled	1/2 cup
Potatoes, sweet or yams	1/4 cup
Rice or grits-cooked	1/2 cup

Vegetable Group

The vegetables in this food group have very few calories and have more fiber, potassium, magnesium, vitamin A, C, folic acid than other food groups. A serving is one cup raw or 1/2 cup cooked.

Asparagus	Mushrooms	Summer squash
Beets	Okra	Tomatoes
Broccoli	Onions	Turnips
Brussels sprouts	Green peas	Winter squash
Cabbage	Red peppers	Zucchini
Carrots	Greens:	Spinach
Watercress	Chard	Lettuce
Cauliflower	Radishes	Cress
Celery	Rutabagas	Beet
Collard	Mustard	Cucumber
Sauerkraut	Kale	String beans
Dandelion	Eggplant	Chicory
Escarole, etc.		

Fruit Group

The portion size of the fruits listed below contain about 40 calories and approximately the same amount of potassium, magnesium, vitamin C and carbohydrate. Some have vitamin A. Bananas and watermelon have some vitamin B6. The portion size of the fruits in the first column are 1/2 cup.

Applesauce	Apple 1 sm	Orange 1 sm
Blackberries	Apricots 2 med	Peach 1 med
Blueberries	Banana 1/2 med	Pear 1 sm
Cherries (10)	Cantaloupe 1/4	Plum 1 med
Grapes (20)	Grapefruit 1/2	Strawberries, 1
Grapefruit juice	Honeydew 1/4 cup	Orange juice
Kiwi (2)	Tangerine 1 med	Pineapple
Nectarine 1 med	Watermelon 1/2	Slice 1" thick
Pineapple juice	Raspberries	

Fat Group

The portion size of the foods below have about 45 calories in fat. The butter fats have vitamin A. The vegetable oils have vitamin E. Vitamin A has been added to margarine.

Avocado 2 tsp	Mayonnaise 1 tsp
Butter, Margarine solid 1 tsp	Seeds 1/2 tbsp
Oil or Cooking fat 1 tsp	Hot dog 1/3
Bologna,	Pepperoni, etc. 1/2
Bacon crisp,1 slice	Nuts 6 small
Cream 20%, 2 tbsp	Olives 5 sm oz
Cream 40%, 1 tbsp	Peanut Butter 1/2 tbsp
Cream cheese, 1 tbsp	Sausage 1/2 oz
Sour cream 1 tbsp	Salad dressing 1 tbsp
Sausage link 1/2	

Some groups share nutrients. For instance, the *Meat* and *Milk* Group share protein, phosphorus, niacin, and B12. However, the Meat group contains zinc, iron and copper which the Milk Group does not have. The Milk Group contains calcium and riboflavin, which the Meat Group does not have. Because of its lack of iron, cheese is not a substitute for foods from the Meat Group.

The *Vegetable* and *Fruit* Groups both contain potassium, magnesium, vitamin C and fiber (not strained). Foods in the Vegetable Group contain very little carbohydrate but they are high in carotene (vitamin A) and folic acid. Whereas, foods in the Fruit Group are high in carbohydrate and lack folic acid. A few orange fruits, like cantaloupe, contain some carotene.

The *Starch* Group like the Fruit Group contains foods high in carbohydrate and fiber. The Fruit Group does not have the B vitamins which the Starch Group does.

The *Fat* Group contains foods that are high in fat but low in other nutrients. The Meat and Milk Group contain some foods that are high in fat. Two are steak and cheddar cheese, respectively.

Vitamins work with the Macro-Nutrients

Vitamins are co-enzymes which work as a team with other nutrients to create an action. You will note that vitamins and minerals do not work alone. They depend on having enough energy from the macro-nutrients and on the minerals to act as their co-factors. Vitamins are divided into water and fat soluble vitamins. The water soluble are vitamin C and the B vitamins. The fat soluble are vitamins A, D, E and K.

Water Soluble Vitamins

Vitamin C is an essential water soluble vitamin which cannot be stored or synthesized. The average person needs to consume about 60 mg a day or one half cup of orange juice or strawberries or melon. The best source of vitamin C is fruits and vegetables.

Vitamin C works as a team with co-factors (minerals), vitamin A, and fat and protein. The vitamin C in fruits and vegetables is ascorbic acid, which increases the acidity of the stomach. The acidity of the stomach prepares calcium from milk, iron and zinc, from the Meat Group and magnesium from the Fruit and Vegetable Groups for digestion and absorption.

Vitamin C acts to reduce the oxidation damage to blood vessels. If the blood vessels are damaged the result will be hemorrhages and gum lesions.

Vitamin C in the meal acts to ward off infections and build up the immune system, to keep the skin smooth and moist, to keep bones strong.

The *B-vitamins* are co-enzymes involved in manufacturing energy from starches, fats and proteins.

Thiamin, or vitamin B1, is a co-enzyme with carbohydrate and other nutrients to create energy. Your best sources of thiamin are whole and enriched grains, watermelon and pork.

Riboflavin, or vitamin B2, along with other nutrients prevents the skin from breaking down, helps the eyes be less sensitive to light, and keeps the intestinal tract healthy. Fifty percent of the body's source of riboflavin should come from the milk products, the rest should come from whole and enriched grains, and green leafy vegetables.

Niacin is so necessary for every action in the body that almost one half of the amount of niacin that the body needs is converted from the amino acid, tryptophan with the help of vitamin B6. Niacin is needed for the liver to break down glycogen and convert it to glucose, to detoxify alcohol, to convert fatty acids to energy. Niacin is needed for the nerves to transmit messages. About a fourth of what your body needs should come from whole and enriched grains. Some can come from nuts, mushrooms, asparagus, and green leafy vegetables. The remainder comes from tryptophan, a protein from foods in the Milk and the Meat Groups or from the breakdown of lean tissue when the cell's protein is converted to glucose.

Vitamin B6 or pyridoxine is a necessary co-enzyme which works with the co-factors, zinc from the meat and milk group and magnesium from the fruits and vegetable groups. The liver uses vitamin B6 to convert amino acids into forms the body cells can use. It uses vitamin B6 to convert tryptophan to niacin and serotonin. Tryptophan needs large amounts of starches. Without enough vitamin B6 and starches, tryptophan can not be converted into serotonin, a neurotransmitter which controls sleep. Vitamin B6 is one nutrient needed to build hemoglobin and is one of the enzymes that controls insulin, the growth hormone and thyroid. Your sources of vitamin B6 are chicken and turkey, fish, whole grain cereals, egg yolks, bananas and potatoes.

Folic acid is necessary to help vitamin B12, copper, iron, and glucose build red blood cells. It is necessary with other nutrients to rebuild cells in the intestinal tract, for cells to multiply, especially during growth and a disease. Folic acid is the co-enzyme necessary to convert phenylalanine to tyrosine. Sources of folic acid are oranges, vegetables, yeast, mushrooms and liver.

Fat Soluble Vitamins

As you may already know from all the publicity, vitamin A and carotene, vitamin E, and vitamin C are vitamins that prevent free radicals from ravaging cells. But again, they cannot do it alone. They need the aid of other macro and micro-nutrients. For instance, fat must be present in the meal for vitamin A and E to be absorbed in the intestinal tract.

Vitamin A and carotene are necessary to attract water from the air and the body, to keep our mucous membranes moist, to keep our immune systems healthy, and to build bones.

Vitamin D is necessary to absorb the minerals calcium, phosphorus, and magnesium when they enter the intestinal tract. These minerals help keep our bones and muscles strong. If vitamin D is not absorbed because of a low fat diet, the body's supply of magnesium is also very low. Muscles will then cramp, become spastic or a rash can erupt on the skin. The best source of vitamin D is sunshine when it converts the cholesterol under the skin. Your other sources are deep water fish such as cod and salmon and the enriched vitamin D milk.

Vitamin E is necessary to prevent the breakdown of cells that carry oxygen to the cells.

Vitamin K is the agent that makes blood clot and prevents death from bleeding. Sources of vitamin K are green leafy vegetables and a special bacteria that the intestinal tract produces

Do Vitamin and Mineral Supplements Make Up for Food?

Vitamins supplements may overshadow the importance of food for some people. I interviewed a first grader once. He told me what he had for breakfast; "I didn't eat anything, but . . . (and here his voice rose expectantly as he looked to me for approval), "I took my vitamin pill."

Each food group contains some micro-nutrients and some macro-nutrients. Food is always the preferred method to provide nutrients to your body. There may be a person who cannot eat foods from a specific food group, either because they are allergic to them or cannot digest them. Without consuming foods from a food group, the body will be missing those nutrients. Therefore, should a person take a vitamin and mineral supplement?

Let's use the Milk Group as an example. The major nutrients which the Milk Group provides are protein, carbohydrate, calcium and riboflavin. Vitamin and mineral supplements can make up for the riboflavin and the calcium, but they cannot make up for the protein and carbohydrate. Therefore, I suggest increasing the serving from the Meat Group one more ounce and the Starch Group one more serving. In this manner, the supplements are just that—supplements *to* the food and not substitutes *for* the food.

Vitamins and minerals are needed in very minute amounts to act as co-enzymes and co-factors in helping macro-nutrients work. Picture the micro and macro-nutrients working together like a football team. If a football player is missing on the field, the others cannot take his place. If there are too many football players on the field, the team is penalized. A deficiency in one vitamin or mineral can produce deficiencies in the others. Overdosing in one can alter and penalize the functions of the others.

In the past two decades, there has been an ever-increasing indiscriminate use of vitamins. Without hard evidence of their need and ingesting more than the body needs, a person can place themselves at risk for some adverse reactions. The higher the dosage, the more the vitamins and minerals can approach a toxic level in the body and the greater the risk for such reactions. Do you know what dose of a vitamin will give you an adverse reaction? The label does not carry a warning nor is there any regulatory agency that ensures the product has what it claims. The supplement lobby fought off regulations and research requirements which the United States Department of Agriculture (USDA) tried to impose. Who would guess that vitamin and mineral supplements which can make a person better can also make them sick? It all depends on the amount taken, the amount in food, their interaction with medications and a person's lifestyle.

The body can ingest more than it needs of vitamins and mineral through foods. Some foods are devitalized through refining and manufacturing techniques and to make up for that loss, many manufacturers add vitamins and minerals to the products to improve their nutrition content.

For instance, years ago, millers refined flour to preserve it. They extracted all the nutrients except the carbohydrate. Researchers discovered that people who consumed white flour products developed deficiencies in several vitamins and minerals. So the government asked the millers to add back thiamin, riboflavin, niacin and iron.

With this model began an avalanche of formulated foods. Today manufacturers may add vitamins and minerals so that the "Nutrition Information" label makes the product look like a natural food or better.

Some manufacturers formulate chemicals to look like, taste like and feel like a real food. But an imitation food product lacks the nutrients we count on from a food group. Without knowing it, you can make a whole meal of fake foods.

Investigate—discover the real versus the imitation by reading the label of "ingredients." The label on the food product lists the ingredients in descending order from the greatest amount to the smallest. Also, compare the words listed under "ingredients" to the words listed in the same product in your recipe book.

Adverse Reactions to Large Doses of Vitamins

If a person believe they should take a vitamin supplement, they should first evaluate their need. Keep a diary of all food intake for one day. Read the "Nutrition Information" on food products which gives the percentages of the vitamins. Total them and compare them to the Recommended Dietary Allowance (See Appendix D). Toxic reactions caused by excess water soluble vitamins that are naturally in foods are unknown. But reactions from supplements is known.

Body cells absorb vitamins through receptors. An excess of one nutrient can smother the receptors, preventing others from entering. Eventually, there will be a deficiency in the nutrient that was shut out.

Below is listed the name of some vitamins, the recommended amount for you as an adult as determined by the Food and Nutrition Board of the National Institute of Sciences, the amount considered an excess and the symptoms of toxicity. If you experience toxic symptoms, just cut back on the dosage. Many of the symptoms can be confused with symptoms of a disease. Experiment by eliminating the supplement for the month. Then begin taking them again and evaluate the reaction.

Toxicity of Water Soluble Vitamins

The body does not store water soluble vitamins, therefore, an excess does not cause the problems that fat soluble vitamins can. But because vitamins compete with other nutrients for the receptors on the cell, even an excess of water soluble vitamins can disturb the balance between the nutrients.

Vitamin C

The recommended dose is 60 mg a day. If you ingest more than 500 mg, your body is receiving more than 500 percent over the recommended dose. Very large doses taken over time may have adverse reactions.

Reactions to a Vitamin C Overdose

- Can prevent the beta cells from producing insulin.

- Blood glucose can rise. People most affected are those with diabetes, hypoglycemia, high blood cholesterol.

- Can precipitate a rise in blood triglycerides.

- Can prevent the absorption of copper resulting in high blood cholesterol and anemia.

- Can change the pH in the intestinal tract preventing enzymes from digesting food, The symptoms are diarrhea, nausea, abdominal cramps and bleeding and/or ulcers. Long term usage of high doses may cause ulcers and cancer.

- A vitamin C tablet not swallowed completely can become lodged in the esophagus and burn the delicate tissues.

- Acidity of chewable vitamin C can erode tooth enamel.

- Can prevent the absorption of vitamin E.

- Can increase the absorption of iron resulting in iron toxicity in the liver, blood and bone marrow and may be a factor in heart attacks.

- Can increase uric acid crystals resulting in kidney stones, joint pain and arthritis.

- Can reduce the fluidity of the blood resulting in a blood clot. May reduce the effectiveness of blood thinning medications.

- Can increase the potency of estrogen.

Mrs. Wiggins had a stroke at an early age. *Coumadin* was prescribed to prevent blood clots. It was a mystery to her physicians why the medication didn't keep the blood thin. She said no one asked if she was taking vitamin supplements, even though her medication's insert carried a warning about vitamin C. She had been ingesting 2000 mg of Vitamin C every day for ten years. Since high doses of vitamin C supplements are known to cause blood clots, the megadose of vitamin C could have been a factor that precipitated the stroke.

Vitamin B1 (Thiamin)

The recommended amount is 1.1 to 1.5 mg. Any amount over that is considered excessive and the following may occur:

- Nervousness, sweating, tremors
- Heart arrhythmias, low blood pressure
- Reduced absorption of other vitamins

Vitamin B2 (Riboflavin)

The recommended amount is 1.3 to 1.7 mg. Any amount over that is considered excessive. Riboflavin is more difficult to absorb in the intestinal tract. If too much is ingested you may experience:

- Itching and a rash
- Paralysis
- Macular degeneration, a disease of the retina

With as little as twice the RDA, and a generic weakness the excess riboflavin causes a build up of lipofuscin, a toxic waste, a fatty build up that invades the retina of the eye cells leading to legal blindness.

Niacin

The recommended amount is 15 to 19 m equiv. Excess niacin can affect the liver and can lead to:

- Flushing of the skin and tingling sensation
- Nausea, heartburn, headache and ulcers
- Increases in uric acid excretion
- Irregular heart beat and low blood pressure
- A rise in triglycerides
- Dermatitis and a rash
- A rise in blood glucose plus, people affected are those with diabetes or hypoglycemia.

If you have these symptoms, cut back because long term use of excess niacin can lead to liver damage and the development of diabetes.

Vitamin B6 (Pyridoxine)

The recommended amount is 1.6 to 2 mg. An excess amount can lead to:

- Numbness and permanent paralysis
- Liver damage
- Parkinson's Disease
- Convulsions in the newborn, if the mother ingests more than 50 mg a day during pregnancy.

Folic Acid (Folacin)

The recommended amount is 180 to 200 mg. Any excess amount can lead to:

- Gastric upset
- Sleep disturbances
- Lethargy, irritability
- Masked B12 deficiency
- Prevents zinc from being absorbed

Toxicity of Fat Soluble Vitamins

Unlike water soluble vitamins which are excreted, fat soluble vitamins can accumulate and build up in the liver and body fat. The antioxidant craze has fueled the flames of the supplement buying frenzy. A survey conducted in 1992 reported that sales of vitamins[37] increased over 1987 by 19 percent and now one third of the population in the United States is taking supplements daily.

Vitamin A

Recommended amount is 5000 I.U. per day for adults. Excess vitamin A accumulates in the body and when it reaches 100,000 I.U. The following symptoms may appear.

- Anorexia and vomiting
- Headaches and irritability
- Spotty hair loss
- Increased pressure in the brain may cause retardation

- Brain damage
- Bone damage and joint pain
- Kidney damage from the accumulation of calcium in the blood
- Dry and scaly skin
- Muscle weakness and fatigue
- Enlargement of the spleen
- Liver damage
- Weight loss
- Diarrhea
- Birth defects, especially cleft palate, if taken in excess during pregnancy

Vitamin D

Recommended is 400 I.U. per day. Ingesting over this amount can lead to:

- Nausea, vomiting, diarrhea
- Excessive thirst
- Weight loss
- Nocturia (excessive urination at night)
- Muscle weakness and fatigue
- Headache
- Irritability
- Kidney damage from the accumulation of calcium in the blood
- Calcium deposits in soft tissue in the body
- Retardation
- Damage to heart, lungs, and tissues surrounding joints
- Death

Vitamin E

Recommended is 10 to 12 I.U. a day. Doses of 60 I.U. per day is over 500 percent. If you experience the following cut back on the dosage.

- Thinner blood
- Bleeding or hemorrhages
- Anemia
- A rise in LDL cholesterol
- Headaches, dizziness, blurred vision
- Fatigue, muscle weakness
- Hypoglycemia, depression,
- High blood pressure
- Flu like symptoms
- Clots and phlebitis
- Degenerative changes in the joints
- Gynecomastia (swollen breasts in men)
- Tumors, breast tumors, painful breasts
- Pulmonary embolism
- Impaired absorption of vitamins A and K.

Vitamin K

Excess intake is rare.

Vitamins And Minerals: An Important Part of a Larger Picture

The body lives on food and food can provide all the nutrients except oxygen and some water. Food contains macro-nutrients and micro-nutrients which work together as they are being digested, absorbed and used by the cells. Without the micro-nutrients, the macro-nutrients would be unable to work and vice versa. Everything works better when the body is in balance and in harmony.

CHAPTER 11

Exercise
Making Fuel Work For You

WHAT does fitness mean to you? Is it the Olympic champion skater, the quarterback on Super Bowl Sunday, the pitcher in the World Series, the basketball players on the winning team, or the number one seed in tennis. Most of us never aspire to become this superfit, but we can become plain fit. A fit person is one who uses food and exercise to stay healthy.

The need to move and to exercise is as important to the body as the need for food, for oxygen, for water and for sleep. Food and exercise go together like bees and honey, sun and green grass, fish in water.

However, more than one-half to three-fourths of the population in the United States do not exercise or do strenuous work to the levels recommended for good health benefits according to Walter R. Dowdle, Acting Director of The Centers for Disease Control and Prevention in 1993.[38] People who do meet the criteria of 30 minutes of aerobic exercise three times a week or manual labor several hours a day do make the food they eat work for them.

Muscles make up a large part of this lean tissue, some 45 percent. Some muscles never stop moving. Consider how many times a minute lungs inhale and exhale, or the heart beats, or the eyes blink.

Every time muscles move they use energy and excrete waste products. The energy sources they use are glucose in the blood, glycogen stored in the muscles, and fatty acids in the blood. The waste products are heat, water and carbon dioxide (See Chapter Notes).

Fat Can Be a Source of Energy

When a person exercises, the muscles work harder and faster and use more energy. You may know that muscles use body fat for energy. But fat does not kick in until you have been exercising aerobically for 20 minutes. And then the amount of fat used is only one percent of the mix the rest is glucose. Fatty acids enter the blood stream from the digestion of fat and from the breakdown of fat pads within the body and under the skin. By walking another 20 minutes, more fats break down and increase the fatty acid ratio to 20 percent of the mix. By walking more than an hour, the fatty acid ratio rises to 40 percent. However, beyond an hour, the ratio of fat to glucose in the mix does not increase incrementally as much. It will never reach 100 percent, no matter how long one exercises or works, because there always must be some glucose in the mix of fuels. The muscles always need glucose. During the first 20 minutes they use glucose from the blood. After that their source of glucose is from conversion of muscle and liver or lean tissue (See Chapter Notes).

Glycogen as a Source of Energy

Glycogen is to the body what starch is to plants. It is stored glucose. When dietary starch is digested in the body, 100 percent is converted to glucose. The glucose enters the blood, is carried by insulin into the liver and muscle cells and stored as glycogen. As the blood glucose drops the liver converts the glycogen back 100 percent to glucose. That's more than can be said for protein and fat. Only 50 percent of glucose can be derived from protein while only five to six percent can be derived from fat.

As you exercise or work hard beyond an hour, less and less glucose comes from liver glycogen than from protein in lean tissue, some of which will be muscle unless you eat some starches. With the loss of lean tissue your blood glucose drops. You experience hypoglycemia, headaches, central nervous system problems and exhaustion. Additionally, the muscles become fatigued and you are at a higher risk for injury.

A similar thing can occur when you starve yourself for just one day. Glycogen stores are depleted. The glucose being produced from lean tissue and body fat cannot replenish liver glycogen. Ketones build up in the blood and potassium, water and lean tissue cells are lost. It takes several days to replenish the glycogen and that will take plenty of starch carbohydrates. If you starve your body episodically, the liver may eventually lose its ability to store glycogen.

Glycogen is gradually depleted during the night when you are sleeping. Doesn't it make sense to eat before exercising in the morning? However, many people have the mistaken idea that they will burn up more body fat if they exercise before they eat. But with glycogen stores low and the need for energy high, lean tissue, including muscle tissue, will be used instead.

Is Sugar a Source of Energy?

If you eat at least 300 calories of foods with some starch and a little protein before you exercise, you will protect your lean tissue. But sugary cereals, sweet coffee cakes or candy bars will not. The sugar stimulates the insulin hormone and blood glucose will drop in about 15 minutes and you will feel very fatigued. In fact, sugar reduces performance by 25 percent. Exercising shortly after a meal reduces blood glucose slowly and insulin is not produced. Exercising after the meal can also reduce blood fats, blood cholesterol and triglycerides.

When to Exercise

How soon after a meal should you exercise? Have you been told to wait an hour? Yes, you should if you have a hiatus hernia or ulcer, heart disease, feel woozy or your stomach churns. You should wait one half to one hour and then the kind of exercise you should do should be walking only. Running and jumping bounces the stomach juices around. Walking after a meal rarely causes any problems. In fact, it may give relief from bloating and discomfort.

As muscle cells work, they break down and need to be rebuilt by calories and nutrients from food. You need to add more calories, the more intensely and the longer you exercise. Running, for instance, uses about 100 to 200 calories more an hour than walking. To maintain your weight, you may need to exercise three to four times a week, for about 30 to 40 minutes each time (See Chapter Notes). If you need to lose body fat, you can exercise 500 calories off daily which for a woman will take about 60 minutes. And for a man about 50 minutes.

If you exercise more than an hour, more calories are needed to prevent using muscle and lean tissue for energy. Meals should include lots of starches, a small amount of protein and some fat. The protein is necessary to rebuild cells that break down during exercise. Some athletes believe they need more protein to build muscle. However, increasing the amount beyond 15 percent has no magical power to make muscles bigger and faster. In fact, extra protein in such products as amino acid powders and formulas can be harmful. They require more water, place a greater load on the kidneys to rid themselves of the waste products, encourage the release of calcium from bone, and place a greater stress on the liver for increased enzyme production. Additionally, extra protein is converted to body fat.

Replenishing Glycogen Stores

Exercise and replenishing muscle and liver glycogen are the two keys to staying fit (See Chapter Notes). In replenishing glycogen there are three phases. First you need to start out with high glycogen stores. Then, if the exercise continues for over 40 minutes, you may need to replenish the gycogen *during and after* exercise. Diluted fruit juices and starchy carbohydrates can replenish glycogen better than foods high in protein, fat and sugar. A sport drink, which has only six to eight percent sugar, may replace some of the blood glucose and fluids during an event but does not replace other nutrients. It is better to save concentrated sugar products such as candy, soft drinks, commercial powdered fruit aides and fruit drinks or drinks with caffeine for after the exercise. Caffeine not only stimulates the insulin hormone which leads to a drop in blood glucose, but it is a diuretic. Soft drinks can produce bloating or diarrhea because they pass through the intestinal tract too fast. Children because of their smaller liver and muscles have less capacity to store glycogen. Children need to eat and drink every 15 minutes while participating in a strenuous sport. A suggestion is graham crackers and diluted fruit juice.

Some people overtrain. When they do, their pulse rate and blood pressure rise. They become anemic. They may lose weight, but the weight is lean tissue. Women may stop menstruating. All of these signs and symptoms are an indication that the person has not been eating enough food in the right combination to keep up with the demand. They are not fit. They are not using their food to keep them healthy (See Chapter Notes).

Is There a Fast Way To Build Muscle?

As people exercise, their muscles grow larger. Additional blood vessels carry the nutrients to the larger muscles. Bones become stronger as the bones respond to the pull of the muscles by becoming more dense and heavier. The added muscles, blood vessels, and bones add up to more lean tissue weight. Men, because they have more testosterone, have an advantage over women in building muscles. But aside from this, building muscles and bone is a slow process that cannot be hurried (See Chapter Notes).

However, impatient athletes may take anabolic steroids. The muscles grow larger, but the bones lag in growth. When strong muscles pull on weak bones, the bones can snap. It is like pulling the string on a bow to shoot an arrow. If the bow is not strong it will snap. Anabolic steroids are potent drugs which can produce many other problems such as mental disturbances, impotence, heart disease and cancer. Perhaps the expectations of an athlete are beyond his or her reach. Each person inherits a specific type of muscle which is better for one sport but not for another (See Chapter Notes).

In one of my nutrition classes were two young men, Bobby and Harry, ages 19 and 20, who wanted bigger muscles and worked out every day. Bobby was taking steroids and following a poor diet. Harry did not take steroids but he followed a meal plan of 3600 calories. At the end of six weeks, Harry gained six pounds of muscle (lean tissue). Bobby gained none. When Bobby saw the results, he told me he quit the steroids and followed the meal plan. In six weeks he gained four pounds of lean tissue.

Many athletes are proud of the fact that their body fat is very low. But too little body fat prevents the production of testosterone, a hormone necessary for building muscles. Additionally, building muscles means challenging them with extra work to grow more cells and then keeping those cells filled with glycogen. Starch carbohydrates can do that (See Chapter Notes). Muscles absorb glucose at a faster rate immediately after exercise and continue to work at a higher metabolism *for the next 24 hours.*

When muscles are not used, their metabolism slows and your muscles only absorb five percent of the available glucose. This is particularly important for overweight people with diabetes who lack good glucose absorption in the first place. As they say, "Use them, or lose them." When they are not used, muscles become flabby.

Unused muscles cannot negotiate stairs easily, or carry your body very far before you need to sit down.

However, it is never too late to build muscles. All it takes is the will to begin. Muscles will return with encouragement, exercise, persistence and patience. People can begin by walking very slowly in their home for ten minutes every day or walking up and down the corridors in a building (See Chapter Notes).

Ten years ago, a man in his late 60's came to me for a diet. He had angina, a disease of the coronary blood vessels which prevents an efficient circulation of oxygen. Pain occurs on exertion but with medication it is bearable. He thought he could not exercise. I suggested he receive permission from his doctor to walk every day. I suggested he start out very, very slowly the first week and only walk for 20 minutes a day, then he could add one minute each week. It took him two months before he could walk a mile in 35 minutes. In four months he lost 25 pounds even though he was consuming 2200 calories divided into three meals and a snack. His doctor allowed him to discontinue the angina medication. At that same time, he began to build an addition to his house. He said to me, "If you had told me *five* months ago that I could build an addition on my house, I would have told you, you are crazy because I have angina and all I can do is sit in my rocking chair and wait to die." Ten years later he is still walking every day and following his meal plan.

Anemia Slows Performance

One cause of the lack of oxygen is the lack of red blood cells (or anemia). Red cells in the blood carry oxygen from the lungs to all cells in the body. Fewer red blood cells means less oxygen is available to the cells and may be a result of bleeding somewhere in the body, by an infection or the lack of nutrients and calories to rebuild cells. Bleeding and infection must be identified and treated and substances such as medication, tea, vitamin supplements that prevent the absorption of iron must be eliminated. Often, to speed the building of red blood cells, people are told to ingest iron supplements. However, iron supplements are not the total solution. Building red blood cells take more than one nutrient and can't be hurried without all 60 nutrients. And ingesting high amounts of iron for too long can damage liver cells. Additionally, while iron is being absorbed, zinc and copper are squeezed out. These three minerals compete for the same carrier to move them across the intestinal tract into the blood stream.

Instead of ingesting iron supplements, a person can rebuild their red blood cells in about a month or six weeks with the right mix of nutrients and calories at each of three meals a day, provided the anemia is nutritionally related.

Supplements

In addition to iron, many people believe they can enhance their physical performance by taking liquid or powder supplements. Research has found that vitamin and mineral supplements have little or no benefit at enhancing physical performance.[39] For instance, niacin is sometimes used in supplement form by athletes. But large amounts of niacin prevent the release of fatty acids from body fat stores, not a desired state. Muscles need body fat as an alternative fuel when people are involved in any kind of endurance work such as working at the office or in a factory or running in a marathon. In fact, research shows that consuming some fat in the diet helps improve physical performance.[40] That may occur because less oxygen is necessary to convert fat to energy than carbohydrate.

Another supplement that athletes believe they need to use is potassium to replace the potassium lost in sweat. But large amounts of potassium can lead to cardiac arrest. Supplemental drinks are a life saver for those who can't eat, but to balance physical performance, food is better.

Water To Cool the Heated Muscles

Muscles need water. As they work, they create heat that the blood must shunt off to the outer parts of the body, to the skin, where sweat evaporates and cools down the body. When people sweat, they lose weight—water weight (See Chapter Notes).

There is a danger from losing too much water weight. A person who loses seven percent of his or her weight in water can die. A football player who loses five to seven pounds in a game will find it difficult to continue and too tired to care. Blood flow is reduced. Less glucose, oxygen and nutrients can reach the cells. Muscles become fatigued including the heart and lung muscles. Less sweat is excreted. Body temperature rises. Blood becomes warm, and can result in heat damage to the body cells. The consequences can be heat cramps, heat exhaustion and even a deadly heat stroke. Less blood flow to the kidneys means waste products are not excreted. Instead, they accumulate in the blood, becoming toxic to the cells.

The goal then is to prevent loss of water weight. However, tiredness and dehydration can sneak up on a person because during exercise the thirst hormone lags behind the body's actual need for water. To prevent dehydration, drink plenty of water before, during, and after exercising or working in a hot environment (See Chapter Notes). Of course if you swim, your body is being kept cool. But you still need to drink a cup of water every half hour.

People who have diarrhea and consume alcohol or caffeine and a diuretic medication are losing water. They should be careful about exercising and ask permission from their physician. Other medications may produce intestinal distress. If they do, they should take them an hour before exercising to prevent bleeding or other side effects which can become exaggerated during exercise.

It was believed at one time that the sodium needed to be replaced. But research[11] has revealed the opposite. Sodium concentrates in the blood by the kidneys. Therefore, adding sodium as in salt tablets or sport drinks only complicates the fluid balance. What is needed is plain and simple: water—and make it cold.

The Rewards of Exercise

The response by the body to exercise and to the right treatment with nutrients is very gradual. Eventually, the heart muscle becomes stronger and slows it's beat. The muscles of the blood vessels become stronger and contract strongly as they propel the blood along. Blood pressure returns to normal. There is an increase in the number of blood vessels carrying more oxygen to the cells. The lungs process oxygen with less effort. Energy increases. You may discover you are less stressful, less anxious, less depressed. Your skin becomes more taut, has more color and is moist. Your blood tests show normal blood triglycerides, LDL cholesterol and HDL cholesterol. Exercise allows insulin to carry the glucose into the liver and muscle cells, a benefit for those with Type II Diabetes. For women, exercise can reduce the production of estrogen.

Less estrogen means less body fat, less premenstrual tension and less menstrual cramps.

How can you tell if your muscles are stronger? You may not have lost any weight, but your clothes fit better. Your stomach may be flatter (See Chapter Notes). When you are measured, you have lost body fat and gained a few pounds of lean tissue. The food you eat, instead of being deposited as body fat, is being used by your muscles for energy and enlarging them. Exercise is easier and you can exercise for an extended time. You are able to climb a flight of stairs without sitting down.

"Use it or lose it." Years ago, a person said to me, "You must be a tennis player." I asked, "How can you tell?" He answered, "Your right arm is bigger than your left." I gave up tennis a few years ago. Now my right arm has become the same size as my left.

What Fitness Mean to You

It means:

- More energy
- A heart that is fit, beats strongly, about 60 to 65 beats per minute at rest.
- Lungs that are fit and breathe 14 respirations per minute and can inhale more oxygen at rest.
- The ability to sleep soundly for seven to eight hours.
- The body is receiving enough calories and nutrients from food to protect its lean tissue and it is receiving enough for exercise.

It also means:

- A normal body composition of 16 to 18 percent body fat for women and 16 to 20 percent for men.
- Bones that are strong and dense.
- A good immune system which translates into less colds and less infections.
- Normal blood cholesterol and blood triglycerides without medication.
- Normal blood pressure without medication.
- Less insulin.
- A calm body and mind that can deal with stress.

- A good self image.
- A mind that can think clearly.
- A better sex life.
- A body that can climb four flights of stairs.
- An intestinal tract that is neither bloated, cramped or irregular.
- Joints that move easily and well.

It means eating three daily meals of food with enough calories and nutrients to support lean tissue, It also means drinking eight glasses of water, walking or exercising aerobically for 30 minutes three times a week or engaging in manual labor several hours a day.

Can fitness be accomplished? Many people have with patience, motivation, perseverance, determination, encouragement and support from others. It may mean changing your lifestyle a little but once the benefits are realized, most of us become converts. As someone once said, "Exercise can add life to our years and years to our life."

Chapter Notes:

1: Muscles always use glucose to produce energy even when they burn fat. Therefore, for the long haul, glycogen, the source of glucose, must be stored in muscles and the liver. The larger the muscles and the liver, the more glycogen that can be stored. A small liver can store 280 calories while a large liver can store 600 calories. Small muscles can store 1200 calories but with training the muscles can enlarge and store 2000 calories.

2: To train for an event, the muscles must be kept fully replenished with glycogen. It may mean letting them rest every third day and the day before an event, to allow the muscles to fill with glycogen. It takes 20 hours of rest for the glycogen to fully replenish muscle stores. Otherwise, if the muscles are exercised every day, they never have a chance to completely be replenished. Calories, as many as 3000 or up to 6000 calories during training may be needed. Some of the meals can include some sugar sweets to meet the carbohydrate need.

3: Exercise has three phases: endurance, stretching and strengthening. Walking can be an endurance exercise, especially if you walk more than 20 minutes. About five to ten minutes after you start your muscles are warm enough for you to stretch them. The arms, legs, back and front muscles should be stretched slowly. Each stretch should be held for a count of ten then relaxed. Stretching exercises should be done at least three times a week. Many fitness places can instruct you on the correct procedure. Swimming is an excellent way for you to warm up the muscles, to stretch and to push against the resistance of the water. It's even better for those with arthritis or heart problems. Water supports the body and with the body in a horizontal position, the heart pumps more blood with each beat. It doesn't need to pump blood up hill like it does for walking or other upright exercises.

To strengthen muscles, you can add weights. Fitness clubs have equipment and supervision that can strengthen muscles. At home without the machines, you can devise your own. For the arms, you can start with a one pound can or weight in each hand then walk. When you can walk with the one pound can with ease, you can graduate to two pound cans and as you feel like it add more pounds. For the legs, you can fill a sealable quart size plastic bag with enough dirt or sand to weigh a pound. After draping the bag over your ankles and then over your heels, you can raise and lower each leg ten times. You need to repeat this exercise three times a week. When you can do this exercise with ease, you can add another pound of dirt to the bag and repeat the exercise. More weight can be added as long as you are at ease. The exercise should be repeated only ten times each session, not more. When you exercise aerobically, you need to slow your pace and a cool down for the last three to five minutes. If you stop abruptly your blood pressure can rise and you may feel dizzy. Drinking a cup or two of cool water should follow. If you take a shower afterwards, make it warm water, not hot. It is advisable not to step into a hot tub or a spa. Results will be slow but, with persistence, you should see a big difference in about two months.

4: Some people are better at one sport than another because of the type of muscles they inherited. Muscles come in two sizes— the short fast twitch muscles and the long slow twitch muscles. People who have predominately short fast twitch muscles are good at wrestling, being a lineman on a football team, or playing ice hockey because they can exert a burst of energy without oxygen. Exercise without oxygen is called anaerobic. People who have predominately slow twitch fibers have long legs and arms and are good as endurance runners and swimmers. This kind of exercise is aerobic. The muscles use more oxygen.

5: If you are just starting to exercise, you can gradually build up the strength of your muscles, including the heart muscle. Walking is an easy exercise. You can start slowly and only walk for about ten minutes the first day. Then you can add a minute each day or every other day until you are up to 30 minutes. If you add music with a great beat it will make the exercise more enjoyable. If your leg muscle becomes painful or burns, you should slow down and allow the lactic acid to clear out. Lactic acid is a substance that builds up in a muscle because it is unable to rid itself of carbon dioxide or has not received enough oxygen.

Either the muscles in your heart are too weak momentarily to pump the oxygen to the leg muscles and/or your chest muscles are too weak to inhale enough oxygen to meet the demand. But if you continue walking, more blood vessels will be added and your heart muscle will be stronger. You will be able to exhale more carbon dioxide. Then you will have fewer episodes of lactic acid build up. You may have heard that trainers sometimes massage the muscles of athletes after an event in an attempt to increase circulation and make the blood carry the left over lactic acid to the liver where it is converted to glucose. Pain also can occur if the muscles are cold. Muscles need to be warmed up in the beginning. Walking very slowly and then gradually increasing the intensity should warm them up in about five minutes. Warm muscles can absorb more oxygen and expel the carbon dioxide better than cold muscles.

6: The body needs to have plenty of water for *two* hours before an event. People should drink two cups fifteen minutes before and then 2/3 of a cup of water every ten minutes during the event. Immediately after the event, they should drink two cups of water for each pound that they have lost. If they have lost a great deal of weight, it may take from 12 to 24 hours to rehydrate the body.

8: "Pinch and inch." With the thumb and forefinger the fat can be pinched up just above either hip bone. Measure it. More than an inch of fat suggests the body has too much fat.

Exercise & Protect Your Body	Before	During	After
Protect your Glycogen Stores			
Adults and children:			
Eat starch and a protein food about 300 calories	30 to 60 min.		
Eat starch food and diluted fruit juice		Every 30 min.	Within 15 min.
Diluted fruit juice		Children every 15 min.	Children every 15 min.
Protect Water Reserves			
Drink water	2-4 cups	1 cup every 10 min.	2-3 cups
Diluted fruit juices		1 cup	1 cup
6 to 8% sugar drinks		1 cup	1 cup
* Ingest any required medications one hour before exercising to prevent intestinal distress.			

CHAPTER 12

Dirt In The Fuel Tank

FOOD, a most precious commodity which has the potential to keep us healthy, also has the potential to make us sick. Food can harbor invisible dirt, bacteria and other contaminants, which can enter the body's "fuel tank" at any time and disrupt its operation. Two thirds of all food borne illnesses originate in restaurants and food processing plants, the other one third comes directly from the home kitchen. Food-borne illnesses kill 9000 people a year. Those most at risk are the people who are undiagnosed, untreated, or have poor immune systems.

People have become increasingly more complacent about food-borne diseases in the last 50 years. They may rely on the health department to keep their sources of food clean or they rely on antibiotics to kill off the bacteria. These antibiotics however, are losing their power. Even the newly-developed antibiotics, we are being told, will only be effective for a few years, making sanitation and vaccination among the preferred methods of prevention.

Our bodies can resist most bacteria and toxins which enter through our mouth, skin or lungs. Each of us has a liver and immune system which, if we are well-nourished, can ward off infections and toxins. Even so, it may not be enough. The more unfortunate may suffer coma and death. Even the healthiest liver and the toughest immune system can be overwhelmed by toxins from food poisoning or bacteria that grows on food or in water. Anyone who has had food poisoning most likely can attest to its sudden onset of vomiting, diarrhea, and fever. Additives, preservatives and metals such as lead also can compromise the liver and immune system too.

The liver and immune system can't protect us without a little help. Be vigilant and learn not to overwhelm your body. Take care of food once it enters your home. Choose restaurants and foods that are clean and practice the sanitation rules. You will have less illness, less absenteeisms from work and school, more enjoyment from life and fewer doctor bills.

Research has shown that bacteria needs the same four conditions to stay alive and grow that humans do: warmth, moisture, oxygen and food. Bacteria grow best in the temperature zone between 40˚ to 140˚ degrees Fahrenheit. So foods can be kept hotter or colder than this temperature range. They can be kept dry. The air can be exhausted and the food or beverage sealed against the deteriorating effects of oxygen. Food can be kept clean and bacteria prevented from entering in the first place.

Five rules that you can use to prevent infection from food-borne diseases are:

- Keep foods clean.
- Keep hot foods hot-over 140 degrees Fahrenheit.
- Keep cold foods cold-under 40 degrees Fahrenheit.
- Cook foods thoroughly.
- When in doubt, throw it out.
- Seal foods against oxygen.
- Drink safe water.

Keep Foods Clean

Hands have the four conditions under which germs grow. They are warm and moist, and can be covered with substrate on which germs can grow.. They have oxygen. Hands are the greatest carrier of the invisible germs.

Germ growth can be blocked. Wash your hands. Wash them before, during and after food preparation. Children, too should learn to routinely wash their hands.

Hands can carry germs from dirty to clean utensils. You wouldn't put your fingers in other people's mouths. Why place dirty fingers on the dishware from which people eat from or inside glassware from which people drink or pick up silverware by the eating end of the handle?

Utensils, dishware and glasses can grow germs if they sit dirty long enough. Once they are washed in hot soapy water, the germs perish. Air drying for an hour before you store them away is better than wiping them with a questionably clean towel. If you have a dishwasher, you should rinse the food off first. Silverware should be stacked in the basket with the handles up so that you do not touch the eating ends when you remove them. Add the sponges and brushes to the dishwasher too and rinse the towels and dishrags in diluted bleach.

Hands can cross-contaminate foods. When you prepare raw foods such as raw meat, poultry products, seafood, chicken, turkey, eggs, fish or red meat, the bacteria from them will coat everything it touches. You should wash your hands with hot soapy water before preparing cold foods such as lettuce, breads, fruits, and cheeses.

Keep Cold Foods Cold

Refrigerators are a great invention. They can keep foods safe until you eat them. They keep bacteria from growing by reducing the moisture, oxygen and temperature. The temperature in the refrigerator is kept at 40˚ degrees Fahrenheit and a fan keeps the moisture low. Keeping the refrigerator door closed as much as possible not only will reduce the amount of air entering but also save on electricity. Yet, bacteria can still grow; it just takes a little longer. A refrigerator that is too full of food means restricted air flow and increased moisture. The result is more mold, bacteria and contaminated food. Spoiled food means wasted money and illness. Instead, an inventory of the contents should be taken every week and meals planned around one-day-old leftovers. "The First foods in should be the first foods out." "If in doubt about a food, throw it out." "Don't keep leftovers over two days."

The refrigerator itself can be a problem. Bacteria can grow on the walls, the shelving, the drip tray and the drawers. Washing with baking soda every few months can remove the bacteria. While cleaning, manufacturers suggest the refrigerator be left on to save the extra electricity it takes to cool down a warm refrigerator. They also suggest you take everything out first. After washing they suggest you rinse and dry the inside and the outside of the food containers before returning them to the refrigerator. The food being returned to the refrigerator should be checked for mold. Notice the emphasis on drying everything to reduce moisture. If the refrigerator has a drain, you can remove the plug and pour warm water and baking soda into it. To make the refrigerator more efficient, manufacturers suggest the condenser coils be vacuumed at least twice a year.

Keep Hot Foods Hot-Over 140 Degrees

Most bacteria in foods can be killed by cooking the food thoroughly at a high-heat setting. However, once foods with protein start to cool down, they enter the danger zone-140˚ down to 40˚ Fahrenheit. The longer the food remains in this danger zone, the more potent the bacteria become. For instance, food left for an hour or two, such as on a counter to cool, at 90 to 100˚ Fahrendeit can grow bacteria so potent it can make a person deathly ill. Not only does the bacteria grow fast, but the quality and the taste of the food deteriorates. The trick then is to flash-cool the food. What better way than to use the gas or electricity that runs the freezer and refrigerator? The colder the environment the faster it will cool. The thicker the food and the tighter it is covered, the longer it takes to cool and the more moisture it retains. Using a shallow container and covering the food an hour later with plastic wrap or aluminum foil is safer.

If you want to reheat leftovers, the reverse process is used. Flash heat it. The leftover food should go directly from the refrigerator into the oven or microwave and the gas or electricity will heat it up. It should not be removed until it is steaming and bubbling. If you just want to heat up a portion of the leftover food, use a clean spoon to dish out a portion into a clean container. The remainder should be refrigerated immediately. Frozen foods should be thawed in the refrigerator, the microwave or oven, not on the counter. Thawing at room temperature is a sure invitation to bacteria to take up residence and ruin the taste.

If hot food is taken to a picnic or potluck meal, bacteria may come along unless the hot food is kept at 200 degrees in a insulated or electrically-heated container. Some people use burners under the pan or dish. Cold foods such as mixed salads and cream filled pastries can be kept cold with ice packs or dry ice in an insulated container. If camping, protect food from flies, bees, mice and bears! To be on the safe side boil, cook or peel the food.

To assure that your home is a safe haven from food-borne disease, ask yourself the questions in the Chapter Notes.

Now that you know how to prevent bacteria from growing in your food, how do you know there isn't bacteria already contaminating what you buy?

Shopping For Food

Since few of us grow our own wheat, fruits and vegetables, or raise animals for meat and milk, we depend on the farmers, the food processors, the manufacturers, the distributors, the grocery stores, and the restaurants for food. Think about this: Never in the history of man have so many people been allowed to handle another's food before it is eaten. Because of these developments, in America the United States Department of Agriculture (USDA) and the Food and Drug Administration (FDA) are providing us with the most marvelous and the safest food system in the world. Still, we are ultimately responsible for our own health. This takes wisdom when we purchase food.

Some of the following questions may help you when you buy food:

- Do the clerks in the bakery or delicatessen wear plastic gloves when they parcel out your bread, rolls, sliced cold cuts and cheese?

- Do you check for cracks in the eggs? Bacteria can enter the cracks and grow.

- Do you buy milk, apple cider or honey that is pasteurized?

- Do you read labels for the ingredients, not just for the nutrition information?

- Do the people who make up your sandwiches at restaurants wear plastic gloves?

- Do you refrigerate your cold food purchases immediately after you bring them home from the market?

- When you prepare food at home, are you tempted to lick the bowl or your fingers when you prepare batter and cookie dough which contains raw eggs? Better to wait until it is cooked. High heat kills off most bacteria if the food is cooked thoroughly.

Dining Out

The creation of the fast food-restaurant phenomenon has reduced many people's responsibility for meal planning and sanitation. How many people wash their hands before eating food from a drive-in restaurant? Fortunately most of the food is wrapped in paper which you can use to keep your unclean fingers off the food. Do you watch to see how waitresses or waiters handle the dishes, glassware and silverware from which you will eat? Does your restaurant have a "sneeze" shield over the salad bar? Is there ice under the cold food and steam coming up from under the hot food? Is there a clean utensil in each dish? Most restaurants are inspected by the county health departments. You, however, are the ultimate inspector.

Frying food is how many restaurants meet the health rules. Flash heating of food kills bacteria and the food can be served hot before the bacteria has a chance to grow. However, the fat in which the food is fried can be a problem. How often is it changed? Black bits stuck to your fried food may mean the frying oil has not been changed recently. Black bits in the fat cause the fat to oxidize and deteriorate. Deteriorated fat means free radicals are released and free radicals weaken your immune system. Vegetable oils in their natural state are protected from oxidation by their content of vitamin E. However, once the oil is heated, vitamin E is destroyed. The frying may kill bacteria, but it can create other health problems.

Purchasing Foods

When buying foods at the grocery, you might want to look for the label which lists the "nutrition information," ingredients and the expiration date. You may find that many of the ingredients listed on the label are not familiar to you or are unrelated to any ingredient from a recipe of a food you may bake or cook. You recognize vinegar, citric acid, salt and/or sugar, additives which have been used for years and have been declared safe. But there are many others which have been added every year. Some of them are: preservatives, anti-caking agents, emulsifiers, thickening agents, moisturizers, bleaching agents and dough conditioners (See Chapter Notes for others). You may not recognize the names, but you can be reassured that each new substance that is added to our food supply has been approved by the FDA and the USDA. We appreciate the additives which keep our food safe and free from bacteria and mold, but we don't appreciate additives which affect us negatively and are only added to enhance the flavor or color.

For instance, people do have allergic reactions to additives. The reactions can range from a runny nose to death. The people who are at the greatest risk for a reaction are those who are allergic to other substances, are malnourished or have a poor immune system.

One of the preservatives to which many people react is the class of sulfites. The symptoms are wheezing, difficulty in breathing, vomiting, hives, diarrhea, abdominal pain, cramps, dizziness and/or headaches. Sulfites became famous a few years ago when it was reported that 20 people had died from ingesting them. Sulfites are added to alcohol, wines, beer, drugs, cosmetics and underarm deodorants to preserve and prevent oxidation. They are used to prevent fruits and vegetables from browning. But since the reported deaths, the FDA and the USDA have asked restaurants not to use them for rinsing lettuce, mushrooms, bananas and apples and other fruits and vegetables. They are allowed in the other products. However, if it is in a food, it must be listed under "ingredients."

Norma, a patient of mine, had lost a great deal of weight from bronchial spasms. She coughed all day and all night. She was down to 85 pounds and had no energy. In reviewing her history, she told me that her ophthalmologist had prescribed eye drops to prevent the advancement of glaucoma. In researching the medication, I read in the Physician's Desk Reference that an adverse reaction to the eye drop may be bronchial spasms. She reported this discovery to her physician who prescribed a different eye drop. In the meantime, I provided her with a diet high in fat and calories to help her gain weight, to improve her breathing and give her more energy. Within a week, she was not coughing. Both eye drops contained the same medication, but the original contained bi-sodium sulfite and the replacement did not. She then experimented with foods and discovered that whenever she ate a food with sulfite, she coughed.

Another preservative is toluene. It is listed as BHT or butyl hydroxyl toluene and is added to wheat products and the packaging of products with wheat. It is also found in markers, gasoline, tar on the roads, paint, nail polish, underarm deodorant.

Marilyn, a nurse, was working in the emergency room helping to set a broken leg when she fainted. In researching the cause, she discovered that the casting material contained toluene. After that, everytime she was unknowingly subjected to a whiff of toluene, she passed out. A year later, she developed lupus, an auto-immune disease, and she had no energy to play her beloved piano or to work. She asked me to help her build up her immune system.

Her history revealed that because she was always fighting her weight, she regularly skipped meals and ate too few calories. She did not realize that she reduced her immune system. To strengthen her immune system, she avoided toluene, increased her calories and ate food every few hours. Her energy came back and she was able to play and teach the piano for an hour at a time.

With more and more people reporting problems with toluene, some manufacturers are omitting it from their cosmetics, but it is still added to food as BHT.

Another preservative added to foods is the class of nitrites/nitrates. They reduce the amount of bacteria that can grow on bacon, ham and cold cuts. However, nitrites/nitrates can change in the body to a cancer causing agent-nitrosamines if foods with vitamin C are not included in the meal. Would you have guessed that when you drink a glass of orange juice at breakfast with your bacon, or have a bacon, lettuce and tomato sandwich you are preventing the formation of nitrosamines in your body? Because of the threat of nitrosamines, some manufacturers are adding two antioxidants, alpha tocopherol (vitamin E) and vitamin C to the nitrites/nitrates. Remember oxygen allows more bacteria to grow. An antioxidant prevents it.

Other substances are added to improve the appearance or taste of food, medications or beverages are colors, flavorings and flavor enhancers. Most of these additives must be proven safe by the FDA and USDA which lists them on the GRAS (Generally Regarded As Safe) list. Of all the colors originally introduced, only seven remain. However, there is still one color, Yellow No. 5 or tartrazine, on the

GRAS list which can cause a reaction in people who are allergic to aspirin. It is now listed as yellow No. 5 under "ingredients."

A flavor enhancer to which some people react is monosodium glutamate (MSG). MSG is a known agitator which can temporarily paralyze nerve endings and in severe cases can result in a high blood pressure crisis which may lead to death. MSG is discussed in Chapter Five.

There are other chemicals that enter the food supply of which we may be unaware because they are used in the feeding of animals and are not listed as additives. It is possible that they can leave a residue which can lead to health problems. They are difficult to track. For instance, flours and other foods are bleached with chlorine to kill off bacteria and to make them more appealing in color. Bleached paper goods used in the packaging of food has dioxin which can migrate to food and make some people ill. Benzene and hexane are sometimes used to extract oil from plants. They are derivatives of gasoline and cause cancer if ingested in large amounts. Irradiation which sterilizes and kills bacteria is used to lengthen the shelf life of some foods. Potatoes and onions are often irradiated to prevent sprouting and deterioration. However, the USDA and the FDA have assured us that no radiation is left in the food. Antibiotics, hormones and other materials which are added to the feed for the animals raised for food can cause problems. The antibiotics added to animal feed can cause an allergic reaction when a person eats the meat. Could this be a reason that bacteria are becoming resistant to antibiotics? One of the latest scares is Mad Cow Disease in England which made the beef dangerous to humans.

Drink Safe Water

In addition to food, the body needs water. Water can be in the form of fruit juice, fruit drinks, decaffeinated soft drinks, decaffeinated tea or coffee. What do you drink? Hopefully, it is water. When you buy commercially-produced drinks check and make sure they are sealed tight. Once air enters, so does bacteria, better to drink it up, refrigerate it or throw it out.

Most people drink the water from the tap in their house or from fountains. The water from lakes, rivers and reservoirs is safer to drink than the water from wells. Even though it may become contaminated by water runoffs from various places, surface water has more opportunity to be cleansed by sunlight, aeration, and plants than the water that remains underground.

Wells are more of a hazard, especially if they are near waste dumps and landfills, underground storage tanks and other chemicals or junk buried underground. These hazardous wastes enter the ground water which seeps into the underground aquifers and underground rock formations where sun and air cannot cleanse them. If your water comes from wells, test it for contaminates.

To destroy bacteria, public water is treated with chlorine. However, chlorine does not rid the water of hazardous wastes, rust from corroded pipes, lead and other heavy metals or dirt which leaks through the cracks of the piping leading to our homes.

Lead Poisoning

Lead can enter the water in the home if the water is softened. The softener can dissolve the lead in the soldered pipes. But today, plastic piping is being used. Plastic piping also eliminates the problem of rust corroding pipes.

Even though some people question the plastic, it is still the better alternative, since ingesting lead produces serious irreversible mental and physical problems, including weak wrists, learning disabilities, decreased growth, hyperactivity, impaired hearing, and brain damage. Because it is difficult to excrete, it can remain in the body causing damage for years.

The U.S. Government has attempted to reduce the public's exposure to lead by ordering it removed from gasoline and lead-based paints. However, lead can still be present in the paint on old houses. Lead is in the dust at the side of the road from the fumes of the old leaded gasoline and can be carried into the home on shoes and clothes. A person working in construction, demolition, with batteries, or in a radiator shop should change their clothes before going home.

Lead is in the printing ink on newspapers and plastic bags. How many people use newspapers to start a fire to broil their food? If you turn plastic bags inside out, the lead in the printing will come in contact with your food. If you keep wine or acidic fruits or fruit juices in cut lead glass bowls or carafes, the lead can be leached out. Originally, cans holding foods were soldered with lead. Now they are welded shut or stored in glass. The amount of lead in pottery made in the United States is regulated and safe. The United States has no control over the lead content of products made in other countries.

You can keep yourself and your children from absorbing the lead from unsuspecting sources if enough calories and nutrients are consumed at each meal so that the liver can process toxins. Less lead is absorbed in the body if you eat foods with fat, zinc and iron from the Meat Group and calcium from the Milk Group. Research has shown that poisoning occurs more in growing children and in those who are malnourished or ill.

To prevent the ingestion of lead from water, attach a filter or buy bottled water. Bottled water is regulated by the FDA. Some of it has been disinfected with ozone rather than with chlorine. Some remove the impurities by carbon filters, reverse osmosis, ion exchange or by distillation. For more information, call the EPA's Safe Drinking Water Hot Line: 1-800-426-4791.

Children should be tested for lead poisoning. If they or you are found to have lead poisoning, a physician may prescribe vitamin C and calcium phosphate supplements to increase the excretion of lead. For more information about lead poisoning, call the National Lead Information Center: 1-800-532-3394.

The time and energy it takes to care for and feed your body is worth more than your wealth. Remember, your health is your wealth.

Chapter Notes:

1: To assure yourself that your home is a safe haven from bacteria which can grow on food, you can take the following test. The questions are similar to those which the county health departments use when inspecting restaurants and food processing plants. You receive a score of five points for each Yes. A score of 65-70 means you receive the Nutrition Safety Award. A score of 40-45 means you receive a Caution Citation Award. A score of 20 or below means your family better eat elsewhere.

Do you sanitize dishrags, sponges, brushes
with chlorine to kill germs?   ____

Do you wash pots, pans, dishes, utensils, cutting boards
and counters with hot soapy water immediately after using?   ____

Is your refrigerator stuffed with food?   ____

Is the temperature of your refrigerator below 40 degrees?   ____

Do you clean your refrigerator with baking soda every month?   ____

Are there any moldy foods in your refrigerator or cupboards?   ____

Are there any insects running around in your food storage places?   ____

Do you keep hot food above 140 degrees?   ____

Do you cool hot foods in the refrigerator?   ____

Do you thaw frozen foods in the refrigerator or microwave?   ____

Do you refrigerate cold foods immediately after purchase?   ____

Do you cook beef, fish and poultry until it is done?   ____

Do you pick up the silverware and the utensils by their handles?   ____

Do you carry glasses and bowls on their bottoms? Edges?   ____

                                                          Total   ____

CHAPTER 13

Coping
Mechanics To Protect Your Fuel Supply

COPING means adjusting to change—changes which occur within your body or in your environment. It means dealing with and attempting to overcome problems and difficulties. When it comes to eating to overcome health problems, there are a myriad of obstacles.

An obstacle may be the messages you hear. Which one should be followed? In today's profit-oriented society it is difficult to separate the "chaf from the wheat." There's a nutrient for every medical problem, a diet for every nutrient, and a professional for every diet. Learning to cope with failing health or just figuring out how to have a healthy and happy life, becomes confusing with all the mixed messages. Every day there is a new theory, a small piece of the puzzle, but one which is made to seem like a very large piece. What message should you trust?

Finding a professional to help you is the first step. Would you try to fix your car without a mechanic or build a house without an architect or fix the plumbing without a plumber? Don't try to fix your nutrition problem without a Registered Dietitian.

A dietitian can help you overcome some of the obstacles. Many others have traveled this road before and you can learn from their experiences. Your best strategy the first week or two of a new diet is to cook your own meals at home and learn how to put the meals together.

One of the first obstacles is shopping for foods. Learn to make a list and to avoid temptation. Eat before going to the grocery store. Become aware and more investigative. You may discover that the product which comes with the free gallon of milk doesn't fit in with your meal plan. Learn how to distinguish real food from the imitation. You may discover that trading additives for natural food is not always the right choice, despite all the advertising to the contrary.

You discover that buying basic foods lends itself to new cooking opportunities. New cooking opportunities take organization and planning. Planning meals for tomorrow and buying foods ahead of time has its positive side when you are hungry or rushed for time. You discover you are less anxious about what you will eat or serve your family for breakfast, lunch and dinner.

Another obstacle is traveling. If you go by car it is easy. You can pack your own food and water. If you go by air, you may need to carry your food. If a meal is to be served, you can call ahead and ask the airline to prepare your food for you. If you go on a cruise, you can ask the cruise headquarters to prepare your special meals.

If you go to a hotel, you can call ahead or meet with the chef or the person who supervises the restaurant staff and ask if they can prepare your food. If you go to a restaurant, you can call early in the day and ask if they can prepare your food. Many restaurants have become accustomed to and welcome accommodating people who are following special meal plans. But they need to know early in the day. If you fail to call ahead, make sure to choose a safe food once you are at the restaurant. Some possibly safe choices are plain broiled chicken or meat without sauces, baked potato, canned fruits and cooked vegetables. Many restaurants will substitute fruit for French fries or potato chips.

Another obstacle is your job. If you have a stressful, high-paced job, one that does not allow much time for lunch, you may want to carry a brown bag lunch. A lunch with a sandwich or two, a piece of fruit, some vegetable sticks and milk or cheese sticks can provide enough calories and nutrients for the next five hours.

Many people agree that making it through the work day with little or no food is a disaster waiting to happen. An inadequate fuel supply can lead to depression, mood swings, lethargy, and motivational breakdown—all conditions that people in fast-paced working environments may fail to recognize. Feeding the body regularly can make the difference between failure and success.

A breakfast and lunch with a healthy snack midway through the morning or afternoon will help you maintain optimum fuel levels and prevent your blood from becoming thick. Thick blood does not move through and supply the fuel to your brain and throughout the body as well as one that is normal.

Without such planning, mindlessness replaces reason. Famished people tend to stop anywhere to eat, including fast-food restaurants and drive-ins on the corner where the menus are often loaded with foods that are deep fried. Haste and hunger can equal candy bars, diet soft drinks or other foods missing in nutrients and not suitable to your new health plan.

You learn some defensive strategies. You use a diary to track your body's responses to foods, meals, medications, non-food substances (See Appendix D).

Another defensive strategy is to eat at the table. Eating and enjoying the companionship of another may be an incentive to slow down your eating and allow more time for you to chew your food, to lay down your fork and sip on water. By extending the meal to twenty minutes, the hypothalamus can tell you that you are full. It's also amazing how food tastes better and how you remember that you ate.

Parties are a fun way to get together with your friends. Don't let the new eating plan or diet prevent you from going. You can always fortify yourself by eating your food before you leave home. Or you can take your food with you.

Following a new food plan means changing your old habits. Your biggest motivation to change will come after you have adhered to the plan for a few weeks and see a difference in how you feel. Your enthusiasm will grow as you discover coping skills you did not know you had. You are less stressful, sleep better, have more energy, and have progressively-less physical problems. Of course, you need to recognize that failure is part and parcel of a nutrition plan. If you fail you can always go back. It's like going up two steps and down one.

Learning to cope means learning how to protect your lean tissue. The result is not only a reduction in symptoms of medical problems but a loss of body fat. When the focus is on saving lean tissue, it changes the way you look at health. Learning to cope also means reducing stress, and one of the first steps is finding someone qualified to help, setting priorities, exercising, eliminating potentially-harmful substances, organizing, playing, and enjoying.

Your overall goal is finding a way to consistently eat enough calories and nutrients to protect your lean tissue. The key is planning for tomorrow before it arrives. You will find you can solve compromising dietary situations and they will pay off. No one can predict when that will be, how your body will react, or when or if you will return to normalcy. You will eat for the health of it and be better than before, because now you can cope.

CHAPTER 14

Finding A Qualified Professional

WHAT is your 80-year health plan? Does it include a meal plan based on your lean tissue weight? Does it include an exercise plan? Does it include other regimes which can keep you healthy (See Health Guidelines in Appendix)? The foods you choose day-by-day are basic to your health. But your body may develop obstacles which can interfere with how well your body digests, absorbs and uses food. If those obstacles are not overcome, what you eat can become your enemy.

Whether it is for a problem or you just want to be healthy, you need to eat. A Registered Dietitian who has the skills to design meals can help you choose foods to lessen your distress. A Registered Dietitian is trained in how and where in the body foods are digested, absorbed and used, and how diseases change all this.

Registered Dietitians, also known as nutrition counselors, work in consort with other health-care professionals. They are equally qualified to design meals for weight management and general nutrition as they are competent to design nutritional regimes for numerous medical problems. They can help with choices of foods to lessen unexplained symptoms or lessen the impact of a disease that has already been diagnosed (See Chapter Notes for list of special problems and diseases that need nutrition counseling).

Nutrition is as important a consideration in the treatment of people as medical care. Registered Dietitians can make the difference between fast recovery in any disease state or continued illness.

Registered Dietitians (RDs) are the health-care professionals with the most extensive training in nutrition. To become a RD one must fulfill four criteria: be a graduate of an accredited baccalaureate degree program in dietetics, nutrition, food science or food systems management, complete either an accredited internship program or a postgraduate degree combined with an internship program, pass the Registered Dietitian examination conducted by The American Dietetic Association (ADA) and finally, maintain their RD certification with the ADA by completing a certain number of continuing education courses every five years. Beyond that about 40 percent of the 65,000 registered dietitians in the United States have gone on to obtain their master's degree, making them among the most well educated of the allied health professionals.

In many states Registered Dietitians are the recognized nutritionists and are certified or have a license. Some people think of Registered Dietitians as nutritionists which they are. However, there is a distinction between the two names. There are no set qualifications for a person to become a "nutritionist." A nutritionist's training and education can range from being a Physician/Nutritionist Certified by the Board of the American College of Nutrition, to a person who simply sends in a required fee to a diploma mill. From this mill, they receive a certificate stating that they are a "Nutritionist."

To locate a Registered Dietitian who can counsel you, you can call the American Dietetic Association 1-800-877-1600 or turn to the yellow pages of the telephone directory. You may find them in private practice or employed by a hospital.

Physicians often refer patients to a Registered Dietitian, as do psychologists, cosmetologists, pharmacists, dentists, other allied professionals and friends. For reimbursement from an insurance company, you may need a prescription from your physician. Ideally, the prescription will provide details of the diagnosis, pertinent laboratory data, medications, and physical findings. Third-party reimbursement for nutrition counseling varies with insurance carriers and for a specific coverage.

Take your spouse, child, parent, friend, or relative to your appointment with the Registered Dietitian. (For one of my appointments, I asked the mother to bring all the people who fed her child. 12 people showed up).

At the first appointment, the dietitian usually requests a general health history, dietary history, medical history, and information regarding physical activities, physical environment and general lifestyle.

Health history includes major medical events in the person's life. Dietary history can include a food diary recorded over several days, eating patterns, food preferences, food purchases, schedules, vitamin and mineral supplements. Medical history includes the results of laboratory tests and prescribed and over-the-counter drugs.

Along with weight, the dietitian measures you to find the ideal body fat and lean tissue. From those measurements, the dietitian calculates the calories and nutrients needed, then analyzes your 2 or 3 day diary of your food intake with the use of a computer program. The dietitian identifies problem areas of nutrient and calorie deficiencies and excesses.

After the completion of current and historical data, the dietitian translates the diet prescription into a practical meal plan. Critical to the counseling process are the setting of realistic goals, suggestions on how to purchase and cook food, recipes, eating out, time management, encouragement and support.

Visits with a registered dietitian may vary in length and number and the charges vary slightly from one region to another. The initial appointment may be one to two hours with follow-up appointments, 20 to 40 minutes. The follow-up appointments help uncover problem areas, provide additional counseling, support and praise for the person's progress and accountability. Follow up appointments may be for a few weeks to several years. Travel, special occasions, and holidays pose considerations about which dietitians can offer sound advice.

Food may be your friend or your enemy. A Registered Dietitian can help food become your friend and health mate.

Chapter Notes:

1: Special areas of advice and consultation by Registered Dietitians are from general nutrition to medical nutrition therapy. The areas they cover are cancer, diabetes, heart disease, gastrointestinal, malabsorption disorders and hiatus hernia, food intolerances, weight management, pregnancy, (normal or problem), malnutrition, high blood pressure, high blood cholesterol, food allergies cachexia, and infant and child nutrition. Also surgery (pre and post-operative advice), chronic or recurring infections, hypoglycemia, anorexia and bulimia. Others include arthritis, celiac disease, kidney disorders, liver disease, lung disease, sports/athletic performance and body building.

APPENDIX A

DIETARY GUIDELINES FOR ALL AMERICANS*

THE Surgeon General, the American Heart Association, The National Cancer Institute, and the National Academy of Sciences recommend the following:

1. Eat a variety of foods.
2. Maintain a healthy weight. Balance food intake with physical activity to avoid gradual weight gain. For those who wish to lose weight, the recommended rate of weight loss is 1 to 2 pounds per week.
3. Choose a diet low in fat, saturated fat and cholesterol. Limit total fat to 30% of total calories. Limit saturated fat to 10 percent of total calories, and dietary cholesterol to 300 mg per day.
4. Choose a diet with plenty of vegetables, fruits and grain products. Choose 5 or more servings of vegetables and fruits and 6 or more servings of starch foods.
5. Use sugars only in moderation.
6. Use salt and sodium only in moderation. Limit sodium to 2.4 grams (2400 mg) per day.
7. If you drink alcohol beverages, do so in moderation.

* Taken from the Surgeon General's report on nutrition and health, *Nutrition Today*, September/October, 1988, pg. 22.

GUIDELINES TO A HEALTHY LIFE

My guidelines for eating differ from the Surgeon General's only that my guidelines are specific for each meal, and are not based on a day's intake of food.

1. Choose a food from each of the six food groups at each of the three meals in quantities to protect lean tissue cells. This is a "balanced" meal. All of the vitamins, minerals, proteins, carbohydrates and fats are present in the amounts that the body needs and uses. Provide whole milk for children, two percent milk for adults.

For Children:	**For Adult:**
Age 6-8 500 Calories	Women: 500 to 600 Calories
Age 8-10 600 Calories	Men: 700 to 800 Calories
Age 10-16 700 to 800 Calories	

2. Divide meals into equal number of calories.

3. Allow no more than 4 1/2 to 5 hours between meals.

4. Eliminate beverages with caffeine and artificial sweeteners.

5. Choose foods and beverages with little or no sugar. A good yardstick is to consume not more than a teaspoonful of sugar per year of age up to a cap of 15 teaspoons (Adults should consider alcohol as sugar, 1 ounce = 15 teaspoons).

6. Choose real foods with little of no processing and as close to their natural state as possible. Read labels. If you do not know what the word means, find out before you buy the product. Additives in our foods now number over 3000.

7. Eliminate vitamin and mineral supplements. They counter the delicate balance between nutrients and the digestive process.

8. Drink 8 to 10 glasses of liquid a day-preferably water.

9. Sleep 7-8 hours (for adults) in a 24 hour period and 10 to 12 hours (for children).

10. Exercise every day to keep bones and muscles fit. A combination of anaerobic and aerobic exercise will provide the stress that bones and muscles need.

11. If you drink alcohol, do so in moderation. Recommended is no more than 2 drinks a day (8 oz wine, or 24 oz of beer or 3 oz of distilled spirits). Pregnant women should avoid alcohol.

SUGAR CONTENT IN PRODUCTS

The cap on sugar intake per day has been set by the Surgeon General's Office in the Dietary Goals for the United States of 1979 and again in 1989 or 10 percent of the total calories:

For Adults:	**For Children:** (1 tsp per age)	
20-24 tsp	0-5 yrs	0-5 tsp
-	6-10 yrs	6-10 tsp
	11-15 yrs	11-15 tsp
*The smaller the child, the less sugar.		

SUGAR CONTENT			
Beverages	**Sugar tsp**	**Candy**	**Sugar tsp**
Nestle's Quik 2-3 tsp	4 1/2	Chewing Gum 2 sticks	1
Kool-Aid, Tang 8 oz	7 1/2	Cough Drop 2	1
*Soft Drinks 12 oz	10	Lifesaver 2	1
*Fruit Drinks 8 oz	10	Starburst Fruit Chew 1	1
*Choc. Milk 8 oz	12	Bubble Gum 1 pc	2
*Shake 10 oz	12	Peanut M&M 14	3
Fruit Cocktail 1/2 cup	5	Choc. Bar w/ Almonds 1 oz	3
Dairy		Snickers 1 oz	3
Low-Fat Choc. milk 1 cup	3	Mars Bar 1 oz	3
*Fruit Yogurt 8 oz	12	Hershey's Milk Choc. 1 oz	3
Frozen Yogurt 8 oz	8	Plain M&M's 31	4
Pies		Reese's Peanut Butter cup	5
Fruit Pies 4.6 oz	4	Cotton Candy 1 cone	5
Coconut Custard 4.6 oz	4	Jelly Beans 10	7
Choc. Cream 4.6 oz	7 1/2	*Hard Candy 1 pc	10
Lemon Meringue 4.6 oz	8	*Lollipop 1	10
Pecan 4.6 oz	12	*Carmels 1	8
Desserts		**Cakes**	
*Brownie 2" sq	6	Crumb Coffee Cake 3.5 oz	3
Danish Pastry 2.3 oz	1 1/2	Eclair with Icing 3.5 oz	3
Doughnut Plain 1.6 oz	2	Cupcake Plain 2 1/2 diam	3
*Pop-Tart 1.8 oz	3	Cupcake with Icing 2.3 oz	5
*Choc. Pudding	4	Sara Lee Choc. Cake 3.2 oz	8
*Jell-O 1/2 cup	4	Strawberry Shortcake 3.8 oz	8
Popsicle 1	4 1/2	Yellow Cake with Icing 3.2 oz	9
Sherbet 1 cup	8	Twinkie 1	5
Ice Cream Sundae 1 cup	10	**Condiments**	
Ice Cream Sandwich 3 oz	4	Catsup 1 tbsp	1/2
*Ice Milk 1 cup	8	Relish 1 tbsp	1
*Canned Fruit 1 cup	8	Honey 1 tsp	1
Cookies		Maple Syrup 1 tbsp	3
Other Kind of Cookies small	1	* Reference: The American Dental Association.	

Whole Grain Cereal (50-120 calories)	Fiber	Sugar	Sodium
Kellogg's All Bran with extra fiber 1/2 cup	14	0	0
General Mills Fiber One 1/2 cup	13	yes	140
Kellogg's Bran Buds 1/2 cup	11	8	320
Kellogg's All Bran 1/3 cup	9	5	4
Health Valley Raisin Bran Flakes 1/3 cup	6	0	185
Kellogg's Bran Flakes 2/3 cup	5	5	0
Kellogg's Fiberwise 2/3 cup	5	5	0
Ewewhon Right Start 1/3 cup	5	0	0
Kolln Oat Bran Crunch 1/3 cup	5	0	0
Barbara's 100% Oat Bran 1/4 cup	5	0	126
Nabisco Shredded Wheat 'n Bran 2/3 cup	4	0	10
Kellogg's Nutri-Grain Raisin Bran 3/4 cup	4	6	0
Kellogg's Cracklin' Oat Bran 1/3 cup	4	7	305
Post Fruit & Fiber Dates & Raisins 1/2 cup	4	8	170
Kellogg's Fruitful Bran 1/2 cup	4	9	0
Kellogg's Raisin Bran 1/2 cup	4	9	200
Post Natural Raisin Bran 1/2 cup	4	9	195
Health Valley Oat Bran Flakes 1/2 cup	4	0	10
Puffed Kashi 1 1/3 cup	3	0	0
Nabisco Shredded Wheat 1 biscuit	3	0	10
Kellogg's Nutri-Grain Wheat 3/4 cup	3	2	170
Weetabix 1 1/4 biscuits	3	2	0
Post Grape-Nuts 1/4 cup	3	3	160
General Mills Total or Wheaties 1 cup	3	3	370
Ralston Whole Grain Wheat Chex 3/4 cup	3	3	190
Nabisco Fruit Wheats 1/4 cup	3	5	15
Quaker Life 3/4 cup	3	5	150
Kellogg's Frosted Mini Wheats 4 biscuits	3	6	5
General Mills Raisin Nut Bran 1/2 cup	3	8	0
Health Vallery Real Oat Bran Raisin 1/4 cup	3	0	4
Grainfields Oat Bran Flakes 3/4 cup	3	0	0
General Mills Cheerios 1 1/4 cup	2	1	330
General Mills Honey Nut Cheerios 3/4 cup	2	10	345

New Morning Oatios 1 1/4 cup	2	0	0
Kellogg's Kenmei Rice Bran 3/4 cup	2	4	0
General Mills Oatmeal Raisin Crisp 1/3 cup	1	8	0
General Mills Wheaties Honey Gold 3/4 cup	1	10	0
Granola and Muesli (90 to 130 Calories)	**Fiber**	**Sugar**	**Sodium**
Arrowhead Mills Maple Nut Granola 1/4 cup	6	0	13
Familia 25% Bran 1/3 cup	5	6	0
Health Valley Healthy Crunch 1/4 cup	4	0	4
Alpen 1/4 cup	3	5	0
Familia 1/3 cup	3	6	0
Kellogg's Mueslix Golden Crunch 1/3 cup	3	10	105
Breadshop Fat Free Granola 1/4 cup	3	0	0
Health Valley Fat Free Granola 1/4 cup	3	0	0
Health Valley Real Oat Bran Crunch 1/4 cup	3	0	4
Rainforest Granola 1/3 cup	0	3	0
Quaker 100% Natural 1/4 cup	2	7	11
Kellogg's Low Fat Granola 1/3 cup	2	8	0
Ralson Muesli 1/3 cup	2	8	0
Nature Valley 100% Natural 1/3 cup	1	6	50
Refined Cereal (90 to 110 calories)	**Fiber**	**Sugar**	**Sodium**
Ralson MultiBran Chex 3/4 cup	4	6	262
General Mills Basic 4 1/2 cup	2	6	0
Post Honey Bunches of Oats 3/4 cup	2	6	0
Kellogg's Corn Flakes 1 cup	1	2	250
Kellogg's Product 19 or Special K 1 cup	1	3	225
Kellogg's Frosted Flakes 1/4 cup	1	11	200
Kellogg's Rice Krispies 1 cup	0	0	305
Kellogg's Nut & Honey Crunch 3/4 cup	1	9	0

* In *Parenting* Oct. 1992, pg. 193-194. A reprint from the Center for Science in the Public Interest (CSPI) *Nutrition Action Health Letter* All product information obtained by CSPI from the manufacturers.

SUGAR CONTENT IN CEREALS (1989)	
PRODUCT	**% SUGAR**
Puffed Rice (QO)	0.1%
Puffed Wheat (QO)	0.5%
Shredded Wheat (N)	0.6%
Corn Flakes (NM) *	0.8%
Wheat Flakes (EW)*	1.1%
Cheerios (GN)	3.0%
Crispy Brown Rice Cereal (EW)*	3.1%
Wheat Chex (RP)	3.5%
Corn Chex (RP)	4.0%
Rice Chex (RP)	4.4%
Kix (GM)	4.8%
Aztec (Ew)*	4.9%
Post Toasties (GF)	5.0%
Corn Flakes (K)	5.3%
Special K (K)	5.4%
Grape Nuts (GF)	7.0%
Super O's (EW)*	7.1%
Rice Krispies (K)	7.8%
Wheaties (GM)	8.2%
Total (GM)	8.3%
Fiber Seven Flakes (HV)*	8.7%
Concentrate (K)	9.3%
Product 19 (K)	9.9%
Oat Bran Flakes (HV)*	11.0%
Buckwheat (GM)	12.2%
Blue Corn Flakes (HV)*	13.0%
Grape Nuts Flakes (GP)	13.3%
40% Bran (GF)	13.0%
Team (N)	14.1%
Life (QO)	16.0%
Oat Bran O's, Fruit & Nut (HV)*	16.0%
Rice Bran Cereal, Almonds (HV)*	16.0%

PRODUCT	% SUGAR
Orangeola, Almond Date (HV)*	17.0%
Fortified Oat Flakes (GF)	18.0%
All Bran (K)	19.0%
Real Oat Bran Cereal (HV)*	19.0%
100% Bran (N)	21.0%
Life, Cinnamon (QO)	21.0%
Country Crisp (GF)	22.0%
Orangeola, Hawaiian Fruit (HV)*	23.6%
Frosted Mini Wheats (K)	26.0%
Fruit and Fitness (HV)*	26.0%
C. W. Post (GF)	28.7%
Raisin Bran (EW)	28.0%
C. W. Post, Raisin (GF)	29.0%
Raisin Bran (K)	29.0%
Cracklin' Bran (K)	29.0%
Golden Grahams (EW)*	30.0%
Fruit and Wheat (EW)*	31.7%
Capt'n Crunch, Peanut Butter (QO)	32.2%
Cocoa Puffs (GM)	33.3%
Trix (GM)	35.9%
Frosted Rice (K)	37.0%
Honey Comb (GF)	37.2%
Alpha Bits (GF)	38.0%
Count Chocula (GM)	39.5%
Capt'n Crunch (QO)	40.0%
Cookie Crisp, Oatmeal (RP)	40.1%
Crazy Cow Strawberry (GM)	40.1%
Quisp (QO)	40.7%
Sugar Frosted Flakes of Corn (K)	41.0%
Cookie Crisp, Chocolate (RP)	41.0%
Lucky Charms (GM)	42.2%
Fruity Pebbles (GF)	42.5%
Cocoa Pebbles (GF)	42.6%

Cocoa Crispies (K)	42.0%
Capt'n Crunch, Crunchberries (QO)	43.3%
Cookie Crisp, Vanilla (RP)	43.5%
Frankenberry (GM)	43.7%
Frosted Rice Krinkles (GF)	44.0%
Corny Snaps (K)	45.5%
Crazy Cow, Chocolate (GM)	45.6%
Super Sugar Crisp (GF)	46.0%
Sugar Corn Pops (K)	46.0%
Raisin Bran (GF)	48.0%
Fruit Loops (K)	48.0%
Apple Jacks (K)	54.6%
Sugar Snacks (K)	56.0%

Key: (EW) Erewhon, (GF) General Foods, (GM) General Mills, (HV) Health Valley, (K) Kellogg, (QO) Quaker Oats, (N) Nabisco, (RP) Ralston-Purina.

Sugar Content in cereal was analyzed by the United States Department of Agriculture, in 1989.

* Information provided by the company itself, not the USDA.

THE EFFECTS OF CAFFEINE

- Can increase basal metabolic rate.
- Can raise blood pressure and resting heart rate.
- May aggravate fibocystic breast disease.
- Dehydrates the body, is a diuretic and promotes calcium loss.
- Can raise blood glucose and causes the release of insulin-does not help one lose weight.
- Can increase triglycerides.
- Delays fatigue until late in the day.
- May cause headaches, restlessness, and anxiety.
- Reduces the absorption and storage of iron, resulting in anemia.
- May affect fetus or nursing infant.
- Effect on a person depends of size (i.e.) a child drinking a 12 oz. can of cola equals an adult drinking four cups of coffee.

The use of caffeine to speed up body activity affects the pancreas and adrenal glands. Caffeine in large quantities can produce anxiety, depression, even hallucinations, says Psychiatrist Andrew H. Mebane of the Oschner Clinic, who has researched the link between caffeine and psychiatric disorders.[51]

One in 10 adults in America suffers from caffeine-related disorders such as insomnia and headaches. The symptoms can lie dormant for ten to 15 years, giving a message that the stimulant is harmless to the body.

Caffeine affects the central nervous system by delaying fatigue and increasing restlessness. The heart rate, digestive secretions, respiratory and metabolic rates increase. Because caffeine acts as a diuretic, urine output also increases taking with it many nutrients like calcium, iron, magnesium. Caffeine can prevent the absorption and storage of iron. Thus caffeine can contribute to osteoporosis and anemia.

Caffeine can produce short term significant increases in blood pressure. It may cause blood pressure to remain permanently high in some people.

Fibrocystic disease of the breast can be aggravated with caffeine. Many gynecologists recommend elimination of caffeine as a prelude to surgical removal of cysts: the surgery may become unnecessary.

CAFFEINE LEVELS IN DRUG PREPARATIONS:*

There are more than 2000 nonprescription drugs in which caffeine is an additive. It is listed under ingredients.

Product	Caffeine (mg/pill)	Product	Caffeine (mg/pill)
Over the Counter Stimulants		**Cold Preparations**	
No Doz	100	Cenegisic	15
Vivarin	200	Contact	0
		Corban-D	30
Pain Relievers		Dristan Decongest.	0
Advil	0	Drist. A-F Decongest.	0
Anacin, Analgesic	32	Neo-Synephrine	15
Anacin Max Str.	32	Sinapils	32
Anacin-3	32	Triaminicin	30
Cope	32		
Excedrin Extra Str.	65	**In General, the Amount of Caffeine in the Following Types of Products is:**	
Goody's Headache Powder	32		
Midol Original	0	Over the Counter Stimulants	100-200
Nuprin, Aspirin	0	Pain Relievers	0-65
Vanquish	33	Prescription Pain Relievers	0-100
Prescription Pain Relievers			
Apectpol	40		
Darvon Compound	32.4		
Cafergot	100		
Feldene	0		
Migral	50		
Fiorinal	40		
Migralam	100		
Esgic	40		
Soma Compound	32		

Data on caffeine content obtained from the *Physicians' Desk Reference for Nonprescription Drugs*, 1987, and from the *Physicians' Desk Reference*, 1987, and *U.S. Department of Health and Human Services, Public Health Service, Food and Drug Administration, Office of Public Affairs*, 5600 Fishers Lane, Rockville, MD 20857.

CAFFEINE CONTENT

The Surgeon General's office does not mention caffeine, but I recommend drinking or eating as little as possible. *"How much caffeine does it take to get you going in the morning?"*

BEVERAGE	CAFFEINE (mg*)	BEVERAGE	CAFFEINE (mg*)
Coffee (5 oz cup)		**Soft Drinks** (12 oz)	
Drip Method	110	Mountain Dew	54
Percolated	64-124	Mello Yello	52
Instant	40-108	TAB	46
Decaffeinated	2-5	Coca-Cola	46
		Diet Coke	46
Tea (5 oz)		Dr. Pepper	40
1-Min. Brew	9-33	Pepsi Cola	38.5
3-Min. Brew	20-46	Diet Pepsi	36
5-Min. Brew	20-50	RC Cola	36
Sun Tea	2-5	Diet Rite	0
		Sprite	0
Cocoa (1 oz)		Sundance	0
Milk Chocolate	6	Gingerale	0
Baking Chocolate	35	Cream Soda	0
Cocoa Bev. (6 oz)	10	Root Beer	0
Choc Milk (8 oz)	10	Selzer Water	0
		Club Soda	0
		Perrier Water	0
		7-Up	0

* Consumers Union, Food and Drug Administration, National Coffee Association, and National Soft Drink Association.

At least 70 types of soft drinks manufactured by the 12 leading bottlers contain no caffeine. If caffeine has been added to a product, it will be listed under ingredients.

MEAL PLANS FOR REGULAR DIETS

Below are meal plans for 2000, 2400, 2800 and 3200 calorie meals and examples of how to choose foods for those meals.

GENERAL DIRECTIONS FOR FOLLOWING THE MEAL PLANS

- Success in making A MEAL PLAN work is:

Follow The Meal Plan:

Choose foods from the Food Groups in chapter 10. The nutrients and calories in each meal combination work together as they are being digested and used by the cells. Plan meals to be no more than five hours apart. Drink at least 8-10 glasses of liquid-preferably water-over a day. Eliminate these items: Caffeine, Sugar, Alcohol, Nicotine, Vitamin and Mineral Pills, Sugar Substitutes (Nutrasweet, Equal, saccharin), and any medications that are an option.

Exercise:

Exercise aerobically every day for 40 minutes at a time (do not break it up). Exercise after a meal. Aerobics are walking, biking, roller or ice skating, cross country skiing, dancing, swimming, or running. Exercise increases circulation and moves more oxygen into each cell.

PLAN AHEAD:

Plan today for tomorrow. Decide what you will eat and when, and where. Decide ahead of time how you will handle various eating situations. Also, plan today how you will fit exercise into your schedule tomorrow. Enlist a support person.

READ labels and recipes for hidden sources of sugar. SUGAR words are: sugar, honey, syrups. molasses, sucrose, fructose, dextrose, sorbitol, mannitol, zylitol.

READ labels for SODIUM. It is used as a preservative, to flavor foods, or to improve the baking. Some of the sodium words are: salt, baking soda, soy sauce, Worcestershire sauce, baking powder, **sodium** phosphate, mono**sodium** glutamate, di**sodium** sulfate, di**sodium** inosinate, etc.

2000 CALORIES MEAL PLAN

Each meal in this calorie meal plan will have the following **macro** nutrients:

	Grams Per Meal	Percent of the Calories.
Protein	22-26 gms	or 15-16 %
Fat	16-17 gms	or 25-30 %
Carbohydrate	86-87 gms	or 55-60 %
Calories	600 gms	or 28-30 %

BREAKFAST:

1 Oz	MEAT GROUP	1 Egg-poached or boiled
31/2 Servings	STARCH GROUP	1 c Cooked cereal & toast
1-3 Servings	FAT GROUP*	1 tsp Butter
1 Serving	FRUIT GROUP	1 c Strawberries
1/2 Serving	MILK GROUP	1/2 c 2% Milk

LUNCH:

2 Ounces	MEAT GROUP	2 oz Broiled chicken
31/2 Servings	STARCH GROUP	1 Large bun & 1 baked Potato-medium
1-3 Servings	FAT GROUP*	1 tbsp Sour cream or 1/2 tsp Butter or oil
1 Serving	VEGETABLE GROUP	1/2 c Green beans
1 Serving	FRUIT GROUP	1 Apple
1 Serving	MILK GROUP	3/4 oz Cheddar cheese

DINNER:

1-2 Oz	MEAT GROUP	1-2 oz Lean ground round Made into spaghetti sauce
31/2 Servings	STARCH GROUP	1 c spaghetti & 1 slice French bread
1-3 Servings	FAT GROUP*	1 tbsp Salad dressing
1 Serving	VEGETABLE GROUP	Green Salad
1 Serving	FRUIT GROUP	1 c Watermelon
1 Serving	MILK GROUP*	1 tbsp Parmesan cheese

BETWEEN MEALS:

1 Oz	MEAT GROUP	
Or		
1/2 Serving	MILK GROUP	3/4 oz. Mozzarella cheese
And		
1 Serving	STARCH GROUP	English muffin spread With Italian tomato sauce
Or		
1 Serving	FRUIT GROUP	

Nutrition Information:

Protein = 80 gms	**Fat = 54 gms**	**Carbs = 300 gms**

Percent of the Recommended Dietary Allowances for the following leader nutrients:

Sodium ** = 93%	**Potassium = 92%**	**Calcium = 151%**
Iron = 151%	**Vitamin A = 161%**	**Thiamin = 188%**
Riboflavin = 139%	**Niacin = 165%**	**Vitamin C = 367%**
Crude fiber = 910%	**Dietary fiber = 2140%**	

* See Fat Serving

** If your physician recommends that you reduce your sodium intake, you can substitute pasta, potatoes, rice, grits for the breads. Instead of adding salt to foods, you can add chopped vegetables such as celery, parsley, onions, garlic, green peppers, tomatoes (without salt) and herbs. Instead of cheese which is high in salt you can substitute milk or plain cultured yogurt. Instead of commercial salad dressings, you can make your own with lemon juice, oil and herbs. (See recipe) You need a certain amount of sodium in your food every day. And if your kidneys are healthy they produce hormones which adjust to the amount of dietary sodium and maintain a safe level in the blood.

2400 CALORIES MEAL PLAN

The only difference between the 2000 and 2400 calorie meal plan is the 2400 calorie meal plan has one more starch and one more fat per meal.

The macro nutrients for each meal will have approximately:

	Grams per meal	Percent of the calories.
Protein	25-30 gms	or 15-16 %
Fat	19-20 gms	or 25-26 %
Carbohydrate	108-110 gms	or 55-60 %
Calories	600	or 28-30 %

BREAKFAST:

1 Oz	MEAT GROUP	1 Egg-poached or boiled
5 Servings	STARCH GROUP	1 1/2 c Cooked cereal
		3 Slices toast
2-4 Serving	FAT GROUP*	2 tsp Butter
1 Serving	FRUIT GROUP	1 c Strawberries
1/2 Serving	MILK GROUP	1/2 c 2 % Milk

LUNCH:

2 Oz	MEAT GROUP	2 Oz broiled chicken
5 Servings	STARCH GROUP	1 Large bun & 2 baked Potatoes-med
2-4 Servings	FAT GROUP*	1 1/2 tbsp Sour cream 2 tsp Butter or oil
1 Serving	VEGETABLE GROUP	1/2 c Green beans
1 Serving	FRUIT GROUP	1 Apple
1 Serving	MILK GROUP*	3/4 oz Cheddar cheese

DINNER:

1-2 Oz	MEAT GROUP	1-2 oz Lean ground round Made into spaghetti sauce
5 Servings	STARCH GROUP	1 c Spaghetti 2 Slices French bread

2-4 Servings	FAT GROUP*	1 1/2 tbsp Salad dressing
1 Serving	VEGETABLE GROUP	Green Salad
1 Serving	FRUIT GROUP	1 c Watermelon
1 Serving	MILK GROUP	1 tbsp Parmesan cheese

BETWEEN MEALS:

1 Oz	MEAT GROUP	
	Or	
1/2 Serving	MILK GROUP	3/4 oz Mozzarella cheese
	And	
1 Serving	STARCH GROUP	English muffin spread With Italian tomato sauce
	Or	
1 Serving	FRUIT GROUP	

Nutrition Information:

| **Protein = 95 gms** | **Fat = 65 gms** | **Carbs = 360 gms** |

Percent of the Recommended Dietary Allowances for the following leader nutrients:

Sodium = 117%	**Potassium = 110%**	**Calcium = 195%**
Iron = 320%	**Vitamin A = 132%**	**Thiamin = 180%**
Riboflavin = 128%	**Niacin = 165%**	**Vitamin C = 388%**
Crude fiber = 1010%	**Dietary fiber = 2580%**	

* See Fat Servings

** At each meal you have approximately 18 grams of fat to spend. Instead of spending it on sour cream and butter with the baked potatoes at lunch, you can substitute 1 tablespoon of mayonnaise and mix it with boiled potatoes for potato salad.

2800 CALORIES MEAL PLAN

The only difference between the 2000 and the 2800 calorie meal plan is that the 2800 meal plan has 2 more starches and 2 more fats per meal.

The macro nutrients for each meal are listed below:

	Grams per meal	Percent of the calories.
Protein	33-35 gms	or 15-16 %
Fat	23-24 gms	or 25-26 %
Carbohydrate	127-130 gms	or 55-60 %
Calories	840-860	or 28-30 %

BREAKFAST:

1 Oz	MEAT GROUP	1 Egg-poached or boiled
6-7 Servings	STARCH GROUP	1 1/2 c Cooked cereal 3 slices Toast
2-5 Servings	FAT GROUP*	2 tsp Butter or oil

1 Serving	FRUIT GROUP	1 c Strawberries
1/2 Serving	MILK GROUP	1/2 c 2 % Milk

LUNCH:

2 Oz	MEAT GROUP	2 oz broiled chicken
6 Servings	STARCH GROUP	1 Large bun & 2 1/2 med Baked potatoes
2-5 Servings	FAT GROUP*	2 1/2 tbsp Sour cream or 2 tsp Butter or oil
1 Serving	VEGETABLE GROUP	1/2 c Green beans
1 Serving	FRUIT GROUP	1 Apple
1 Serving	MILK GROUP	3/4 oz Cheddar cheese

DINNER:

1-2 Oz	MEAT GROUP	1-2 oz Lean ground round Made into spaghetti sauce
6 Servings	STARCH GROUP	1 c Spaghetti & 3 slices French bread
2-5 Servings	FAT GROUP*	2 tbsp Salad dressing
1 Serving	VEGETABLE GROUP	Green Salad
1 Serving	FRUIT GROUP	1 c Watermelon
1 Serving	MILK GROUP	1 tbsp Parmesan cheese

BETWEEN MEALS:

1 Oz	MEAT GROUP	
Or		
1/2 Serving	MILK GROUP	3/4 oz Mozzarella cheese
And		
1 Serving	STARCH GROUP	English muffin spread With Italian tomato sauce
Or		
1 Serving	FRUIT GROUP	

Nutrition Information:

Protein = 115 gms	**Fat = 77 gms**	**Carbs = 420 gms**

Percent of the Recommended Dietary Allowances:

Sodium = 150%	Potassium = 138%	Calcium = 156%
Iron = 207%	Vitamin A = 164%	Thiamin = 184%
Riboflavin = 117%	Niacin = 150%	Vitamin C = 478%
Crude fiber = 1270%	Dietary fiber = 3410%	

* See Fat Servings

With 21 grams of fat to spend on a meal, you can exchange the sour cream and butter at lunch for 1 1/2 tablespoons of mayonnaise and make potato salad.

3200 CALORIE MEAL PLAN

The only difference in the 2800 and the 3200 calorie meal plan is the 3200 meal plan has 3 more starch servings and 3 more fat servings.

The macro nutrients for each meal are listed below:

	Grams per meal	Percent of the calories.
Protein	35-36 gms	or 15-16 %
Fat	25-28 gms	or 25-26 %
Carbohydrate	145-150 gms	or 55-60 %
Calories	950-980	or 28-30 %

BREAKFAST:

1 Oz	MEAT GROUP	1 Egg-poached or boiled
7 Servings	STARCH GROUP	1 3/4 c Cooked cereal
		5 Slices
2-6 Servings	FAT GROUP*	4 tsp Butter or oil
1 Serving	FRUIT GROUP	1 c Strawberries
1/2 Serving	MILK GROUP	1/2 c 2 % Milk

LUNCH:

2 Oz	MEAT GROUP	2 Oz broiled chicken
7 Servings	STARCH GROUP	1 Large bun & 3 med
		Baked potatoes
2-6 Servings	FAT GROUP*	3 1/2 tbsp Sour cream &
		3 tsp Butter or oil
1 Serving	VEGETABLE GROUP	1/2 c Green beans
1 Serving	FRUIT GROUP	1 Apple
1 Serving	MILK GROUP	3/4 oz Cheddar cheese

DINNER:

2 Oz	MEAT GROUP	2 oz Lean ground round
		Made into spaghetti sauce
7 Servings	STARCH GROUP	2 c Spaghetti & 3 slices
		French bread
2-6 Servings	FAT GROUP*	3 tbsp Salad dressing
1 Serving	VEGETABLE GROUP	Green Salad
1 Serving	FRUIT GROUP	1 c Watermelon
1 Serving	MILK GROUP	1 tbsp Parmesan cheese

BETWEEN MEALS:

1 Oz	MEAT GROUP	
	Or	
1/2 Serving	MILK GROUP	3/4 oz Mozzarella cheese
	And	
1 Serving	STARCH GROUP	English muffin spread With Italian tomato sauce
	Or	
1 Serving	FRUIT GROUP	

Nutrition Information:

Protein = 120 gms   **Fat = 87 gms**   **Carbs = 480 gms**

Percent of the Recommended Dietary Allowances for the following leader nutrients:

Sodium = 135%	**Potassium = 142%**	**Calcium = 200%**
Iron = 391%	**Vitamin A = 159%**	**Thiamin = 179%**
Riboflavin = 115%	**Niacin = 154%**	**Vitamin C = 462%**
Crude fiber = 1290%	**Dietary fiber = 3540%**	

* See Fat Servings

(Note you have about 24 grams of fat to spend on a meal).

Fat servings

The number of fat servings in a meal depends on the amount of fat in the meat and milk group. For a 2000 calorie meal plan, you have about 15 grams to spend at a meal.

A serving from the fat group =	4.0 grams
1/2 c whole milk =	4.0 grams
1/2 c 2 % milk =	2.0 grams
1/2 c skim milk =	0.0 grams
3/4 oz of cheddar cheese =	7.0 grams
3/4 oz mozzarella cheese =	4.5 grams
2 tbsp parmesan cheese =	9.0 grams
1 tbsp of sour cream =	3.0 grams
1 egg =	5.5 grams
1 oz of ham =	4.5 grams
2 oz of steak =	16.0 grams
2 oz chuck beef =	7.0 grams
2 oz lean ground round =	3.5 grams
2 oz pork chop =	18.0 grams
2 oz shrimp =	5 grams
2 oz broiled chicken =	2.0 grams
2 oz broiled or boiled salmon =	4.0 grams
1 tbsp Italian or vinaigrette dressing =	7.0 grams
1 tbsp mayonnaise =	11.0 grams
2 oz filet of beef =	2.0 grams
2 oz pork tenderloin strips =	2.0 grams

You can spend your fat allotment to scramble your eggs at breakfast or you can spend it on cheddar cheese. The fat and other food allotments for a meal must be consumed at that meal and not saved for another meal. At lunch you can spend your fat allotment on mayonnaise and mix 1/2 tablespoon with the starch allotment to make potato salad. Or you can add 1/2 tablespoon of mayonnaise to the meal if you substitute skim milk for the cheddar cheese. Note how much fat is in two ounces of steak and pork chops. It is well over your allotment of 15 grams. Instead you can eat 2 ounces of filet of beef or 2 oz of pork tenderloin strips which are low in fat.

Diets
Calculating Approximate Number of Calories Per Meal

TO calculate an overall caloric intake from foods which also have nutrients, you can use the following formula. These are also listed in the Food Groups in Chapter 10. For each ounce of meat, poultry, fish or one egg there are 75 calories.

For each serving of starch which is approximately 1 slice of bread, or 1/2 serving of other starches there are 70 calories (See list in Food Groups in Appendix).

For each teaspoon of fat, oil, margarine, butter, mayonnaise, 1 slice of bacon, etc. there are 45 calories.

For each 1/2 cup serving of fruit or juice there are 40 calories.

For each 1/2 serving of milk or yogurt, 1/4 cup of cottage cheese or 1/2 ounce of cheese use the figure listed in the chart under the Milk Group. The difference in calories is the content of fat.

For each 1/2 cup of cooked or 1 cup of raw vegetables there are 10-15 calories

For each teaspoon of sugar, ther are 16 calories.

For each ounce of 80 proof alcohol there are 65 calories, (higher proof alcohol contains more calories). For each 12 ounces of beer, there are 100-150 calories For each 4 ounces of wine, there are 80 calories. Liqueurs have more calories per ounce.

"SAFE DIET"

The Safe Diet is for people who have problems with their intestinal tract, bladder or prostrate.

The purpose of a Safe Diet is prevent injuring or irritating the intestinal tract and to rebuild it with enough calories and nutrients. It may take a month or more for the intestinal tract to mend and even longer for it to normalize. The Safe Diet should be adhered to with the goal of no diarrhea or constipation, bloating and gas for one full month. Then a step program to a more normal diet can be instituted.

Substances to Eliminate While on the "Safe Diet"

Spices from seeds, bark or roots. You are allowed to use herbs such as parsley, basil, marjoram, savory, tarragon, etc.

But eliminate the following:

- Alcohol, soft drinks, coffee, chocolate.
- Artificial sweeteners.
- Vitamin or mineral supplements.
- Products with substitute fats or products which have had the fat stripped from them.
- Raw fruits and vegetables.
- All vegetable oils, especially processed oils such as margarines, frying oils, shortening.
- Any food or medication with lactose.
- Untested drinking water.

General Directions for a "Safe Diet"

Choose the plan suited to your caloric need: 2000, 2400, 2800 or 3200 calories Meal Plan as listed on above pages. Choose foods for each meal from the food groups listed below: the Meat, Milk, Starch, Fat, Vegetable and Fruit Groups. Each food group is classified by its major nutrients and caloric content. An example of how to choose foods for a 2000 calorie meal plan is printed below.

All foods should be cooked in purified water and/or butter.

MEAT GROUP

Each ounce from the meat group or equivalent has approximately 75 calories and the same amount of protein, zinc, iron, copper, B12, phosphorus. The white "meats" such as chicken, turkey and fish have less iron and less fat.

Meat and poultry (beef, lamb, pork, liver, chicken, turkey, venison, etc.) — 1 oz
1 Egg
Fish (1 slice 2"x 2" codfish, mackerel, orange roughy, etc.)
Salmon, tuna, crab   1/4 c (if canned in water)
Oysters, shrimp, clams   5 sm
Sardines (packed in water)   3 sm

MILK GROUP

Eliminate milk or products with lactose or whey, imitation cheeses, imitation milks and imitation sour creams.

The size portion of products listed below contain about the same amount of protein, calcium, riboflavin, phosphorus, and vitamin B12. Fat content makes the difference in calories.

Plain yogurt made with a live culture	1 c = 150 cal
Cheeses: white cheddar,	1 1/2 oz = 170 cal
Mozzarella,	1 1/2 oz = 140 cal
Dry Cottage cheese	1/2 c = 100 cal

Vitamin D is needed to absorb the calcium in these products. The best vitamin D comes from the sun. Just expose your hands and face to the sun for 15 minutes a day.

STARCH GROUP

If foods in the starch group contain fat they should be either butter or the kind of fat listed in the Fat Group. Look for products with as few additives as possible.

Each size portion listed below has the same amount of complex carbohydrates, thiamin, riboflavin, niacin and fiber and has 70 calories.

Breads made with butter or no fat	1 slice
Rolls.,look for French or hard rolls with no fat	1 sm
Croissants made with butter	1 sm or 1/2
Bagel or English Muffin with butter or no fat	1 sm or 1/2
Muffin made with butter	2" diam
Cornbread with butter	1 square = 1 1/2"
Cereals cooked	1/2 c
Cereals cold, no nuts or dried fruit	3/4 c
Rice or grits, cooked	1/2 c
Noodles, macaroni, spaghetti cooked	1/2 c
Crackers without oil	2-6
Taco or tortilla shell, no fat or not fried	1 whole
Vegetables: No dry beans, baked beans, split pea etc.	
Creamed corn	1/3 c
Parsnips	2/3 c
Potatoes, instant, powdered or prepackaged.	
Potatoes, 1 baked, 2" diam or mashed	1/2 c
Sweet or Yam Potatoes	1/4 c

FAT GROUP

Each portion listed below is a "safe fat" and contains the same amount of calories (45), fat and vitamin A.

Butter	1 tbsp
Cream, 20 %	2 tbsp
Cream, 40 %	1 tbsp
Sour cream	1 tbsp

Cream Cheese	1 tbsp
Olive oil* (See note)	1 tbsp
Bacon** (See note)	1 slice

*Pressed virgin olive oil contains Vitamin E and is "safer" on some intestinal tracts than other oils. One teaspoon = 45 calories.

**Bacon contains nitrites which may cause a problem

Processed oils such as margarines, corn, soybean, sesame, cotton seed, peanut may be a problem, so eliminate them until your intestinal tract is mended. That means consume no mayonnaise, olives, nuts and seeds. Eliminate processed meats with spices such as hot dogs, bologna, pepperoni, Spam, sausage, etc.

VEGETABLE GROUP

The vegetables listed below have few calories. A portion is 1/2 cup cooked. Each portion has about the same amount of fiber, potassium, magnesium, vitamin A and C, B6 & folic acid.

All vegetables should be cooked, canned or frozen and have only salt (and or butter) added.

Asparagus	Green Peas
Beets	String Beans
Carrots	Summer & Winter Squash
Celery	Zucchini

FRUIT GROUP

The portion size of fruits listed below contain about 40 calories and approximately the same amount of potassium, magnesium, and vitamin C. Orange fruits may have some vitamin A.

All fruits should be cooked or canned without added vitamin C. No dried fruits.

Applesauce	1/2 c	Apricots	2 med
Baked apple	1 med	Nectarine	1 med
Apple juice	1/2 c	Peach	1 med
Canned cherries	10	Pear	1 med
Grape juice	1/4 c	Strawberries	1 c
Pineapple	1/3 c or 2 slices	Pineapple juice	1/3 c

EXAMPLE OF A "SAFE DIET"

2000 CALORIE DIET

BREAKFAST:

2 oz	MEAT GROUP	2 Poached eggs
3 1/2 Servings	STARCH GROUP	2 Slices whole wheat Bread 1 c cooked cereal
2-4 Servings	FAT GROUP*	2 tsp Butter
1 Serving	FRUIT GROUP	1/2 c Applesauce
1/2 Servings	MILK GROUP	1 Slice mozzarella cheese

LUNCH:

2 oz	MEAT GROUP	2 oz White chicken-broiled
3 1/2 Servings	STARCH GROUP	1 Large baked potato
2-4 Servings	FAT GROUP*	2 tbsp Cream cheese
Or		
1/2 Serving	MILK GROUP	3/4 oz White cheddar cheese
1 Serving	VEGETABLE GROUP	1/2 c String beans
1 Serving	FRUIT GROUP	2 Halves canned peaches

DINNER:

2 oz	MEAT GROUP	2 oz Lean ground round Spaghetti sauce w/o tomatoes
3 1/2 Servings	STARCH GROUP	1 1/2 c Spaghetti
2-4 Servings	FAT GROUP*	2 tsp Butter
Or		
1/2 Servings	MILK GROUP	1 1/2 tbsp Parmesan cheese
1 Serving	VEGETABLE GROUP	Peas 1/2 c
1 Serving	FRUIT GROUP	2 Halves canned pears

SNACK:

1 Slice of bread   3/4 oz mozzarella cheese

* See Fat Servings

Nutrition Information:

The fat is increased to 35 percent of the calories as a way to build up the mucous membranes of the intestinal tract.

Protein = 85 gms   **Fat = 74 gms**   **Carbs = 248 gms**

Percent of the Recommended Dietary Allowances for the following leader nutrients:

Sodium = 57%	**Potassium = 78%**	**Calcium = 108%**
Iron = 95%	**Vitamin A = 128%**	**Thiamin = 146%**
Riboflavin = 114%	**Niacin = 153%**	**Vitamin C = 142%**
Crude fiber = 940%	**Dietary fiber = 2860%**	

STEP-UP DIET

After one month without any intestinal problems, one new food can be introduced at a time. If the intestinal tract receives the food with no trouble, then after three days another food may be introduced. If the intestinal tract reacts, then the "Safe Diet" must be followed for a week before another food can be introduced.

Foods here are listed from *least likely* to cause a problem to *most likely*.

Vegetables: raw lettuce, celery, mushrooms, zucchini, summer squash, carrots. Cooked tomatoes, broccoli, cabbage, cauliflower

Fruits: raw kiwi, nectarine, apricots, peaches, strawberries, watermelon, plums, raspberries, cherries, grapes, apples, pears, oranges, grapefruit, melons.

Fats: Mayonnaise, peanut butter, avocado, vinegar and oil dressing.

After about three or four months without any intestinal tract problems, the fat content can be dropped to 25 percent and you can choose a regular meal plan which fulfills your specific caloric need.

GLUTEN-FREE DIET

The gluten-free diet is for adults who have celiac or sprue or are allergic to or cannot digest wheat.

General Directions

Choose the plan suited to your caloric need: 2000, 2400, 2800 or 3000 calorie Meal Plan. For each meal choose from the food groups listed below: the Meat, Milk, Starch, Fat, Vegetable and Fruit Groups. The Starch Group has been modified to eliminate gluten since the person with gluten sensitivity can never eat wheat, barley, rye or oats again. Each food group is classified by its major nutrients and caloric content.

The initial phase of the diet is the "Safe Diet" to allow the intestinal tract to mend.

Products which contain gluten also are listed.

"SAFE DIET" *WITHOUT* GLUTEN

The Safe Diet should be adhered to with the goal of no diarrhea or constipation, bloating and gas for one full month. Then follow the Step-Up program to a more normal diet.

All foods should be cooked in purified water and/or butter.

MEAT GROUP

Each ounce from the meat group or equivalent has approximately 75 calories and the same amount of protein, zinc, iron, copper, B12, phosphorus. The white "meats" like chicken, turkey and fish have less iron and less fat.

Meat and poultry (beef, lamb, pork, liver, chicken, turkey, venison, etc.)
1 Egg
Fish (1 slice 2"x 2" codfish, mackerel, orange roughy, etc.)

Salmon, tuna, crab	1/4 c (fresh not canned in water)
Oysters, shrimp, clams	5 sm
Sardines, packed in water	3 sm

MILK GROUP

Eliminate milk or products with lactose or whey, imitation cheeses, imitation milks and imitation sour creams.

The size portion of products listed here contain about the same amount of protein, calcium, riboflavin, phosphorus, and vitamin B12. Fat content makes the difference in calories.

Plain yogurt made with a live culture	1 c = 150 cal
Cheeses: white cheddar	1 1/2 oz = 170 cal
Mozzarella	1 1/2 oz = 120 cal
Dry Cottage cheese	1/3 c = 41 cal

Vitamin D is needed to absorb the calcium from these products. The best vitamin D comes from the sun. Just expose your hands and face to the sun for 15 minutes a day.

STARCH GROUP

If foods in the starch group contain fat they should be the fat listed in the Fat Group. Read the ingredients on the label. Look for products with as few additives as possible wheat, barley or oats are not allowed.

Each size portion below has approximately 70 calories and the same amount of complex carbohydrates, thiamin, riboflavin, niacin and fiber.

Breads:

Made with corn, potato, or rice flour with butter or no fat	1 slice
Roll, or muffin	1 sm
Cereals, cooked grits, cornmeal or cream of rice	1/2 c
Cereals, cold, corn or rice w/o nuts or dried fruit	3/4 c

Rice	1/2 c
Pasta made with rice, cooked	1/2 c
Rice Crackers w/o oil	2-6
Taco or tortilla shell made of cornmeal, No oil nor fried	1 whole

Vegetables:

No dry beans, baked beans, split peas, etc.	
Creamed corn	1/3 c
Parsnips	2/3 c
Potatoes-baked, 2" diam. or mashed	1/2 c
Potatoes, no processed, powdered or prepackaged	
Sweet or Yam Potatoes	1/4 c

FAT GROUP

Each portion listed here is a safe fat and contains the same amount of calories (45), fat and vitamin A.

Butter	1 tsp
Cream, 20 %	2 tbsp
Cream, 40 %	1 tbsp
Sour cream	1 tbsp
Cream Cheese	1 tbsp
Olive oil*(See note)	1 tsp
Bacon** (See note)	1 slice

* Pressed virgin olive oil contains Vitamin E and seems to be a "safer" oil for some intestinal tracts than others. One teaspoon = 45 calories.

** Bacon contains nitrites which may cause a problem

Processed oils such as margarines, corn, soybean, sesame, cotton seed, peanut may be a problem, so eliminate them until your intestinal tract is mended. That means no mayonnaise, olives, nuts and seeds. Eliminate processed meats with spices such as hot dogs, bologna, pepperoni, Spam, sausage, etc.

VEGETABLE GROUP

The following vegetables have few calories. A portion is 1/2 cup cooked. Each portion has about the same amount of fiber, potassium, magnesium, vitamin A and C, folic acid and vitamin B6.

All vegetables should be cooked, canned or frozen with only salt (and or butter) added.

Asparagus
Beets
Carrots
Celery

Green Peas
String beans
Summer & Winter squash
Zucchini

Lettuce and other greens can be tried raw but without oil.

FRUIT GROUP

The portion sizes of the following fruits contain about 40 calories and approximately the same amount of potassium, magnesium, and vitamin C. Orange fruits may have some vitamin A.

All fruits should be cooked or canned without added vitamin C (no dried fruits).

Applesauce	1/2 c	Apricots	2 med
Baked apple	1 med	Nectarine	1 med
Apple juice	1/2 c	Peach	1 med
Canned cherries	10	Pear	1 med
Grape juice	1/4 c	Strawberries	1 c
Pineapple	1/3 c or 2 slices	Pineapple juice	1/3 c

SUBSTANCES WHICH CONTAIN GLUTEN
OR ARE MADE FROM WHEAT ***

Gluten is in wheat, barley, rye and oats.

Gluten can be in unsuspecting foods so read the label very carefully. Look for wheat fillers, breaded foods, gums, mixes, thickeners, hydrolyzed starch or vegetable protein, malt or malt flavoring, starch, modified starch or modified food starch, vegetable gum.

For more information on-line, type Celiac. ListServ. Fact Sheet on your computer.

Some products which can contain gluten:
- Prepared meats can contain wheat fillers, such as sausages, frankfurter, bologna, luncheon meats, chile con carne and sandwich spreads
- Breaded meats such as Swiss steaks, croquettes, meat loaf, turkey injected with hydrolyzed vegetable protein, canned tuna in vegetable broth
- Cheese products containing oat gums
- Noodles, spaghetti, macaroni, most packaged rice mixes
- Creamed vegetables, canned vegetables in sauce, baked beans, prepared vegetables and salads
- Thickened or prepared fruits, pie fillings
- Cakes, cookies, and pies
- Bread, crackers and breakfast cereals, graham flours, wheat germ, malt, kasha, bulgur, millet, buckwheat, coucous
- Commercial salad dressings
- Canned soups and soup mixes, bouillon

- Malted milk, commercial chocolate drinks
- non-dairy creamers
- Ale, beer, gin, whiskey, vodka distilled from grain
- Ice cream cones, puddings, commercial candies, chewing gum
- Curry powder, dry seasoning mixes, gravy extracts, meat sauces, ketchups, mustards horseradish, soy sauces, chip dips, distilled white vinegar
- The filler in vitamin and mineral supplements

* Roche Products Inc., Manati, Puerto Rico, 00674

** Shils, M.E., and Young, V.R., *Modern Nutrition in Health and Disease,* 7th Ed, 1988, Lea and Febiger Pub., pg. 1588-1586-1591

EXAMPLE OF A WHEAT AND GLUTEN-FREE "SAFE DIET"

2000 Calories Meal Plan

BREAKFAST:

2 Oz	MEAT GROUP	2 Eggs-poached or boiled
3 1/2 Servings	STARCH GROUP	1 1/2 c cooked grits
		1 Corn tortilla
1-4 Servings	FAT GROUP*	1 tsp Butter
1 Serving	FRUIT GROUP	1 c Applesauce
1/2 Serving	MILK GROUP	1 oz Cheddar cheese

LUNCH:

2 Oz	MEAT GROUP	2 oz Broiled chicken
3 1/2 Servings	STARCH GROUP	1 1/2 c Brown rice
2-4 Servings	FAT GROUP*	2 tsp Butter
1 Serving	VEGETABLE GROUP	1/2 c Green beans
1 Serving	FRUIT GROUP	2 Slices pineapple
1 Serving	MILK GROUP	3/4 oz Cheddar cheese

DINNER:

1-2 Oz	MEAT GROUP	1-2 oz Lean ground round
		Spaghetti sauce-no tomatoes
3 1/2 Servings	STARCH GROUP	1 1/2 c Rice spaghetti
2-4 Servings	FAT GROUP*	2 tsp Butter
1 Serving	VEGETABLE GROUP	1/2 c Cooked carrots
1 Serving	FRUIT GROUP	1 c Watermelon
1 Serving	MILK GROUP	1 tbsp Parmesan

BETWEEN MEALS:

1 Oz		MEAT GROUP	
	Or		
1/2 Serving		MILK GROUP	1 c Rice pudding
	And		
1 Serving		STARCH GROUP	1 med Peach
	Or		
1 Serving		FRUIT GROUP	

Nutrition Information

This meal plan has 35 percent of the calories in fat to allow the intestinal tract to mend.

Protein = 76 gms	**Fat = 75 gms**	**Carbs = 266 gms**

Percent of the Recommended Dietary Allowances for the following leader nutrients:

Sodium = 57%	**Potassium = 78%**	**Calcium = 108%**
Iron = 95%	**Vitamin A = 128%**	**Thiamin = 146%**
Riboflavin = 114%	**Niacin = 153%**	**Vitamin C = 142%**
Crude fiber = 940%	**Dietary fiber = 2860%**	

If you have been diagnosed with celiac, sprue or have a sensitivity to wheat, it may take 3 to 4 months before your intestinal tract is mended enough to accept new foods. Carefully introduce one at a time, a raw vegetable, one fruit, or a tsp. of olive oil, allowing 3 days in between each introduction (See note under "Safe Diet"). In about 4 to 6 months you may be able to eat a Regular Gluten-Free Diet with 25 percent of the calories in fat. Choose the caloric level which will support your lean tissue.

An example of a Regular Gluten-Free 2000 Calorie Meal Plan follows:

EXAMPLE OF A REGULAR GLUTEN-FREE DIET

2000 Calories Meal Plan

BREAKFAST:

2 Oz	MEAT GROUP	2 Poached or boiled egg
3 1/2 Servings	STARCH GROUP	1 1/2 c Cooked grits
		1 Corn tortilla
2-4 Servings	FAT GROUP*	1 tsp Butter
1 Serving	FRUIT GROUP	1 c Apple juice
1/2 Serving	MILK GROUP	1/2 c 2% Lactose reduced milk

LUNCH:

2 Oz	MEAT GROUP	2 oz Broiled chicken
3 1/2 Servings	STARCH GROUP	1 1/2 c Brown rice
2-4 Servings	FAT GROUP*	1 tbsp Salad dressing
1 Serving	VEGETABLE GROUP	Salad greens
1 Serving	FRUIT GROUP	2 Slices pineapple
1 Serving	MILK GROUP	3/4 oz Cheddar cheese

DINNER:

1-2 Oz	MEAT GROUP	1-2 oz Lean ground round
		Made into spaghetti sauce**
3 1/2 Servings	STARCH GROUP	1 1/2 c Rice spaghetti
2-4 Servings	FAT GROUP*	2 tsp Butter
1 Serving	VEGETABLE GROUP	Raw carrots

| 1 Serving | | FRUIT GROUP | 1 c Strawberries |
| 1 Serving | | MILK GROUP | 1 tbsp Parmesan |

BETWEEN MEALS:

1 Oz		MEAT GROUP	
	Or		
1/2 Serving		MILK GROUP	1 c Rice pudding**
	And		
1 Serving		STARCH GROUP	1 med Peach
	Or		
1 Serving		FRUIT GROUP	

Nutrition Information

| **Protein= 78 gms** | **Fat= 55 gms** | **Carbs= 300 gms** |

Percent of the Recommended Dietary Allowances for the following leader nutrients:

Sodium = 108%	**Potassium = 85%**	**Calcium = 126%**
Iron = 118%	**Vitamin A = 371%**	**Thiamin = 205%**
Riboflavin = 131%	**Niacin = 162%**	**Vitamin C = 287%**
Crude fiber = 680%	**Dietary fiber = 1140%**	

* See Box 1

** See recipes

LACTOSE FREE DIETS

A lactose-free diet is for anyone who is ill, has had surgery, or is on a medication that upsets the intestinal tract. It is for people who experience bloating or flatulence after drinking milk, or eating ice cream, ice milk, sherbet, frozen yogurt, processed cheeses, legumes or dry beans.

SOURCES OF LACTOSE

Lactose is found in:

- Liquid milk: whole, 1 percent, skim, 2 percent or 2 percent or low fat milk
- Creamy cottage cheese, cream soups and sauces, ice cream, ice milk or sherbet, frozen or flavored uncultured yogurt, custard and puddings
- Dry milk added to such products as chocolate or cocoa beverages or dry soups or sauces
- Processed cheeses, camembert, limburger and brie
- Lactose is added to products as "whey."
- Instant potatoes and other instant products such as ice tea mixes, orange drinks
- Weight reduction formulas
- Caramel candies
- 2000 medications

Avoid legumes such as navy beans, garbanzo beans, pinto beans, kidney beans, etc., because they need the lactase enzyme to break them down. Some times a pinch of ginger in a serving of legumes will prevent bloating and flatulence.

Choose the level of calories which will support your lean tissue. Here is an example of a 2000 Calorie Meal Plan:

EXAMPLE OF A 2000 CALORIE MEAL PLAN

BREAKFAST:

1 Oz	MEAT GROUP	1 Egg-omelet*
3 1/2 Servings	STARCH GROUP	1 1/2 c Diced potatoes*
1-3 Servings	FAT GROUP**	1 tsp Butter*
1 Serving	FRUIT GROUP	1 c Apple juice
1/2 Serving	MILK GROUP	3/4 oz Cheddar cheese*

LUNCH:

1-2 oz	MEAT GROUP	3/4 Chicken tetrazzini*
3 1/2 Servings	STARCH GROUP	1 1/4 c Spaghetti*
		1 Whole wheat roll
3-4 Servings	FAT GROUP**	Fat in the tetrazzini*
1 Serving	VEGETABLE GROUP	1/2 c Green beans
1 Serving	FRUIT GROUP	1 Apple
1 Serving	MILK GROUP	Cheese in tetrazzini*

DINNER:

1-2 Oz	MEAT GROUP	1-2 oz Lean ground round made into meat loaf**
3 1/2 Servings	STARCH GROUP	1 1/2 med Baked potato
3-4 Servings	FAT GROUP*	1 tbsp Salad dressing
1 Serving	VEGETABLE GROUP	Green Salad
1 Serving	FRUIT GROUP	1 Banana
1 Serving	MILK GROUP	3/4 oz Mozzarella cheese

BETWEEN MEALS:

1 Oz	MEAT GROUP	
Or		
1/2 Serving	MILK GROUP	mix 1/2 c Cultured yogurt*
And		
1 Serving	STARCH GROUP	1 c Strawberries
Or		
1 Serving	FRUIT GROUP	2 tbsp Half & half

Nutrition Information

Protein= 75 gms   **Fat= 55 gms**   **Carbs = 300 gms**

Percent of the Recommended Dietary Allowances for the following leader nutrients:

Sodium = 72%	**Potassium = 134%**	**Calcium = 134%**
Iron = 98%	**Vitamin A = 115%**	**thiamin = 154%**
Riboflavin = 148%	**Niacin = 159%**	**Vitamin C = 427%**
Crude fiber = 960%	**Dietary fiber = 2600%**	

* See recipes. The amount of fat at each meal depends on the amount chosen from the Meat and Milk Groups.

Diets And Recipes

Pulmonary Diet

A pulmonary Diet is for people who have breathing or lung problems. The goal of the meal plan is to increase a person's energy with a few extra calories (300) and with foods that produce less carbon dioxide, a waste product which the lungs must exhale day and night. Because fat produces less carbon dioxide than carbohydrate and protein, the percentage of fat calories is increased and the carbohydrate and protein calories are reduced. Fat and carbohydrate are each 42 and 43 percent, respectively leaving 14 percent for protein.

The example below is for a person who normally should eat a 2000 calorie meal plan.

EXAMPLE OF A 2300 CALORIE MEAL PLAN

BREAKFAST:

1 Oz	MEAT GROUP	1 Egg poached or boiled
3 1/2 Servings	STARCH GROUP	1/2 c Hot cereal
		1 slice Wheat bread
3-5 Servings	FAT GROUP*	2 tsp Butter
		1 slice Bacon
1 Serving	FRUIT GROUP	1 c Apple juice
1/2 Serving	MILK GROUP	1/2 Whole milk

LUNCH:

1 Oz	MEAT GROUP	1 1/2 oz Ground sirloin*
3 1/2 Servings	STARCH GROUP	2 med Baked potato
3-5 Servings	FAT GROUP*	2 tbsp Sour cream*
		1 tbsp Sour cream 1 tsp butter
1 Serving	VEGETABLE GROUP	1 c Green beans
1 Serving	FRUIT GROUP	1/2 c Pineapple juice
1 Serving	MILK GROUP	1/2 c Whole milk

DINNER:

1 Oz	MEAT GROUP	3/4 oz Ground turkey*
3 1/2 Servings	STARCH GROUP	2 slice Wheat bread
3-5 Servings	FAT GROUP*	1 slice Bacon & 2 tbsp mayo
1 Serving	VEGETABLE GROUP	Tomato & lettuce
1 Serving	FRUIT GROUP	1/2 c Applesauce
1 Serving	MILK GROUP	3/4 oz Mozzarella cheese

BETWEEN MEALS:

1 Oz		MEAT GROUP	
	Or		
1/4 Serving		MILK GROUP	mix 1/4 c Whole milk **
	And		
3 Servings		FAT GROUP	1/3 c Half & half
	And		
1 Serving		STARCH GROUP	1 c Strawberries 1/2 banana
	Or		
1 Serving		FRUIT GROUP	

* See Choices for Fat Group in Box 1

** See recipe.

Hard to chew foods should be cooked and chopped.

Nutrition Information:

| Protein = 77 gms | Fat = 105 gms | Carbs = 247 gms |

Percent of the Recommended Dietary Allowances for the following leader nutrients:

Sodium = 76%	Potassium = 100%	Calcium = 130%
Iron = 107%	Vitamin A = 93%	Thiamin = 110%
Riboflavin = 116%	Niacin = 105%	Vitamin C = 228%
Crude fiber = 800%	Dietary fiber = 3000%	

General Directions

Two substances increase the production of carbon dioxide even more than starches and protein. They are sugar and alcohol. Therefore sugar and alcohol should be kept to a minimum. If a person desires a sweet, a small amount (1/4 cup) of a high-fat type ice cream is a better choice than yogurt, ice milk, sherbet, candy, soft drinks, cake, cookies, frosting etc. The latter are too high in sugar, too low in fat and lack nutrients needed to rebuild lung cells.

SIX-MEAL-A-DAY PLAN

The following six-meal-a-day plan is for people who have Diabetes Type II, hiatus hernia, heartburn, or reflux. It is for a pregnant woman with gestational diabetes or for people who cannot eat large amounts of food at one sitting. Every two of the smaller meals equals one of the three-meal-a-day plan in nutrients and calories. The first meal begins right after arising. The next meals follow every 2 1/2 hours later and continues until this interval you retire at the end of the day. A serving from the fat group is included at each meal to slow the transit time of the food traveling through the intestinal tract. Choose the number of calories for your meal plan which will support your lean tissue. The example below is for a 2000 calorie meal plan.

EXAMPLE OF A 2000 CALORIE SIX-A-DAY MEAL PLAN

First Meal:

1/2 Serving	MILK GROUP	1/2 c 2% Milk
2 Servings	STARCH GROUP	1 c Cooked cereal
1 Serving	FAT GROUP	1 tsp Butter
1/2 Serving	FRUIT GROUP	1/2 Banana or
		1/2 Unsweetened applesauce

Second Meal:

1 Oz	MEAT GROUP	1 Boiled or poached egg
1 1/2 Servings	STARCH GROUP	1 1/2 Slice wheat toast
1 Serving	FAT GROUP	1 tsp Butter
1 Serving	FRUIT GROUP	1/2 c Orange juice or
		1/2 c Apple juice

Third Meal:

1/2 Serving	MILK GROUP	3/4 oz Cheddar cheese
1 1/2 Servings	STARCH GROUP	1 1/2 Slice bread or
		2 large pretzels
1 Serving	FAT GROUP*	
1 Serving	FRUIT GROUP	Apple or
		1/3 c Unsweetened pineapple

Fourth Meal:

2 Oz	MEAT GROUP	2 oz Broiled chicken
2 Servings	STARCH GROUP	1 med Baked potato
2 Servings	FAT GROUP	2 tbsp Sour cream
1 Serving	VEGETABLE GROUP	1/2 c Green beans

Fifth Meal:

1/2 Serving	MILK GROUP	1/2 c Cultured yogurt**
1 1/2 Servings	STARCH GROUP	5 Graham crackers
1 Serving	FAT GROUP	1 tbsp Half & half**
1 Serving	FRUIT GROUP	1/2 c Strawberries**

Sixth Meal:

1-2 Oz	MEAT GROUP	1 oz Lean ground round
2 Servings	STARCH GROUP	1 1/4 c Spaghetti
2 Servings	FAT GROUP	2 tsp Olive oil
1 Serving	VEGETABLE GROUP	Salad greens or
		1/2 c Cooked carrots

Seventh Meal if needed:

1 Oz	MEAT	
Or		
1/2 Serving	MILK GROUP	3/4 oz Mozzarella cheese
And		
1 1/2 Servings	STARCH GROUP	2 sm English Muffins
Or		
1 Serving	FRUIT GROUP	w/ or w/o Italian Tomato sauce

Nutrition Information

Protein = 75 gms	**Fat = 55 gms**	**Carbs = 300 gms**

Percent of the Recommended Dietary Allowances for the following leader nutrients:

Sodium = 79%	**Potassium = 97%**	**Calcium = 158%**
Iron = 126%	**Vitamin A = 128%**	**Thiamin = 149%**
Riboflavin = 152%	**Niacin = 143%**	**Vitamin C = 232%**
Crude fiber = 800%	**Dietary fiber = 2490%**	

* See Box 1

** See recipes

MEAL PLANS FOR CHILDREN

The meal plans for children outlined next are for 1800, 2200 and 2600 calories. Suggested are the calories for an age level. Note each age level is assigned a different percentage in fat, protein and carbohydrate calories. The younger the child the higher the percentage of fat and the lower the percentage of protein and carbohydrate (See Chapter 4).

1800 Calorie Meal Plan for Children

The 1800 calorie meal plan is for children ages 5 to 7 years of age. The calories are divided into 40 percent fat, 12 percent protein and 48 percent carbohydrate

The macro nutrients for each meal are listed below:

	Grams per meal	Percent of the calories.
Protein	15-17 gms	or 12-13 %
Fat	23-24 gms	or 39-40 %
Carbohydrate	60-66 gms	or 46-50 %
Calories	510-520	or 28-30 %

EXAMPLE OF 1800 CALORIE MEAL

BREAKFAST:

1/2 Oz	MEAT GROUP	1/2 Egg-boiled or scrambled
2 1/2 Servings	STARCH GROUP	1 1/2 c Cold cereal 1 slice toast
2-4 Servings	FAT GROUP*	2 1/2 tsp Butter
1 Serving	FRUIT GROUP	1/2 c Orange juice
3/4 Serving	MILK GROUP	3/4 c Whole milk

LUNCH:

1/2 Oz	MEAT GROUP	1/2 oz Chicken
2 Servings	STARCH GROUP	2 Slice bread
2-4 Servings	FAT GROUP *	4 tsp Butter
1 Serving	VEGETABLE GROUP	1/2 c String beans
1 Serving	FRUIT GROUP	Banana
1 Serving	MILK GROUP	3/4 c Whole milk

DINNER:

1 Oz	MEAT GROUP	1/2 oz Lean ground round
2 Servings	STARCH GROUP	1 c Mashed potatoes
2-4 Servings	FAT GROUP*	4 tsp Butter
1 Serving	VEGETABLE GROUP	Raw carrot strips
1 Serving	FRUIT GROUP	Apple
1 Serving	MILK GROUP	3/4 c Whole milk

BETWEEN MEALS:

1 Oz	MEAT GROUP	
	Or	
1 Serving	MILK GROUP	Smoothie made with 3/4 c Whole milk** & 2 tbsp Half & half
	And	
1 Serving	STARCH GROUP OR	1/2 c Strawberries
1 Serving	FRUIT GROUP	1/2 Banana

Nutrition Information

Protein = 54 gms	**Fat = 80 gms**	**Carbs = 216 gms**

Percent of the Recommended Dietary Allowances for the following leader nutrients as established for this age child by the National Academy of Sciences:

Sodium = 145%	**Potassium = 220%**	**Calcium = 137%**
Iron = 122%	**Vitamin A = 563%**	**Thiamin = 143%**
Riboflavin = 194%	**Niacin = 127%**	**Vitamin C = 307%**
Crude fiber = 730%	**Dietary fiber = 2510%**	

* See Box 1

** See recipes

2200 CALORIE MEAL PLAN FOR CHILDREN

The 2200 Calorie Meal Plan is for children seven to 11 years of age. The calories are divided into 38 percent fat, 14 percent protein and 48 percent carbohydrate.

The macro nutrients for each meal are listed below:

	Grams per meal	Percent of the calories
Protein	23-25 gms	or 13-14 %
Fat	26-28 gms	or 38-39 %
Carbohydrate	6-85 gms	or 47-49 %
Calories	645-680	or 28-30 %

EXAMPLE OF 2200 CALORIE MEAL

BREAKFAST:

1 Oz	MEAT GROUP	1 Egg-boiled or poached
4 Servings	STARCH GROUP	1 1/2 c Cold cereal**
		2 slices Toast
2-4 Servings	FAT GROUP*	3 tsp Butter
1 Serving	FRUIT GROUP	1/2 c Orange juice
3/4 Serving	MILK GROUP	3/4 c Whole milk

LUNCH:

1 Oz	MEAT GROUP	1 oz Chicken
4 Servings	STARCH GROUP**	2 Slice bread
		4 Butter cookies
2-4 Servings	FAT GROUP*	3 tsp Butter
1 Serving	VEGETABLE GROUP	1/2 c String beans
1 Serving	FRUIT GROUP	sm Apple
3/4 Serving	MILK GROUP	3/4 c Whole milk

DINNER:

1 Oz	MEAT GROUP	1 oz Lean ground round
4 Servings	STARCH GROUP**	1 c Mashed potatoes or
		2 Peanut butter cookies
2-4 Servings	FAT GROUP*	3 tsp Butter
1 Serving	VEGETABLE GROUP	Raw carrot strips
1 Serving	FRUIT GROUP	Pear
3/4 Serving	MILK GROUP	3/4 c Whole milk

BETWEEN MEALS:

1 Oz	MEAT GROUP	
Or		
3/4 Serving	MILK GROUP	Smoothie made with
		1 c Whole milk***
		& 1 tbsp half & half

	And		
1 Serving		STARCH GROUP	1/2 c Strawberries
	Or		
1 Serving		FRUIT GROUP	1/2 Banana

Nutrition Information

Protein = 77 gms	Fat = 92 gms	Carbs = 264 gms

Percent of the Recommended Dietary Allowances for the following leader nutrients:

Sodium = 174%	Potassium = 242%	Calcium = 149%
Iron = 144%	Vitamin A = 566%	Thiamin = 145%
Riboflavin = 192%	Niacin = 139%	Vitamin C = 436%
Crude fiber = 960%	Dietary fiber = 2690%	

* See Box 1

** 2 medium size cookies can be substituted for just one serving of starch and one to two servings of fat per meal as long as the rest of the meal is eaten. The nutrients in the meal are needed to process the sugar.
*** See recipes

2600 CALORIE MEAL PLAN

The 2600 calorie meal plan is for children in their fast growth years which may be between 12 and 18 years of age. The calories are divided into 35 percent fat, 14 percent protein and 51 percent carbohydrate.

The macro nutrients for each meal are listed below:

	Grams per meal	Percent of the calories
Protein	26-30 gms	or 13-14 %
Fat	29-30 gms	or 35-36 %
Carbohydrate	96-99 gms	or 49-51 %
Calories	760-780 gms	or 28-30 %

EXAMPLE OF 2600 CALORIE MEAL

BREAKFAST:

1 Oz	MEAT GROUP	1 Egg-boiled or poached
4 Servings	STARCH GROUP	2 c Cold cereal*
		2 slice Toast
2-4 Servings	FAT GROUP*	3 tsp Butter
1 Serving	FRUIT GROUP	1 c Orange juice
1 Serving	MILK GROUP	1 c Whole milk

LUNCH:

1 Oz	MEAT GROUP	1 Oz Chicken
4 Servings	STARCH GROUP**	3 slices Bread
		2 Peanut butter cookies
2-4 Servings	FAT GROUP*	3 tsp Butter

1 Serving	VEGETABLE GROUP	1/2 c String beans
1 Serving	FRUIT GROUP	1 Apple
1 Serving	MILK GROUP	1 c Whole milk

DINNER:

1 Oz	MEAT GROUP	1 oz Lean ground round
4 Servings	STARCH GROUP**	1 1/2 c Mashed potatoes
		3 Butter cookies
2-4 Servings	FAT GROUP*	4 tsp Butter
1 Serving	VEGETABLE GROUP	Raw carrot strips
1 Serving	FRUIT GROUP	Pear
1 Serving	MILK GROUP	1 c Whole milk

BETWEEN MEALS:

1 Oz	MEAT GROUP	
	Or	
1 Serving	MILK GROUP	Smoothie made with 1 c milk***
		& 1 tbsp half & half
	And	
1 Serving	STARCH GROUP OR	1/2 c Strawberries
1 Serving	FRUIT GROUP	1/2 Banana

Nutrition Information

| **Protein = 91 gms** | **Fat = 101 gms** | **Carbs = 330 gms** |

Percent of the Recommended Dietary Allowances for the following leader nutrients:

Sodium = 214%	**Potassium = 309%**	**Calcium = 194%**
Iron = 174%	**Vitamin A = 612%**	**Thiamin = 159%**
Riboflavin = 206%	**Niacin = 144%**	**Vitamin C = 631%**
Crude fiber = 1070%	**Dietary fiber = 3040%**	

* See Note on Fat Choices

** See note under 1800 calorie meal plan

*** See recipes

Children during their teen years may need more calories than 2600. If so, the diet follows the same pattern as the 2600 Calorie Meal Plan with the same percent of protein, the same amount of fruits and vegetables but there will need to be more starch and fat at each meal. However, each meal will contain no more than one cup of milk (2 percent or whole) and no more than 2 ounces from the Meat Group. When the child is fully grown, he or she can follow the adult meal plans which have less fat and more carbohydrate.

* The following are recipes mentioned in the diets

RECIPES

Entrees:
Omelet with Potato
Spaghetti with Beef
Chicken Tetrazzini
Hawaiian Chicken Salad
Poached Chicken Breasts
Starch Dishes:
Reduced Sugar and Fat Raisin Bran Muffins
Brown Rice
Cranberry Bread
Dressings for Salads:
Creamy Dressing for Fruit Salad
Low Fat Buttermilk Dressing
Desserts:
Fruit Smoothie
Fresh Fruit Mix
Peach Cobbler
Apple Crisp
Indian Pudding
Rice Pudding
Low Fat Rice Pudding
Strawberry Cream Dessert

Key to Match the Recipes to the Diet

Lactose Free Diet	LF
Gluten Free Diet	GF
Safe Diet	SAFE
Blood Cholesterol Reducing Diet	CHOL
Diabetic Diet	DIAB
Pulmonary Diet	PUL
Children's Diets	CH

OMELET WITH POTATO AND VEGETABLES

LF, GF, SAFE (without onions), CHOL, DIAB, PUL, CH

Serves 1:

In a frying pan, brown 1 tbsp onions and 1/2 chopped celery stalk in 1 tsp butter for one minute. Add 1/4 c mushrooms and cover for 2 minutes. Add 1 boiled potato diced and 1/4 cup corn. Turn heat down to medium low. Fold in one beaten egg and 3/4 ounce of grated cheddar cheese. Cover for 2 minutes. Serve with a sprig of parsley, fruit and dry toast.

Nutrition Information for One Serving

Calories: 407
Protein = 18.5 gms   **Fat = 17 gms**   **Carbs = 45 gms**

Percent of the Recommended Dietary Allowances for the following leader nutrients:

Sodium = 11%	Potassium = 21%	Calcium = 30%
Iron = 20%	Vitamin A = 22%	Thiamin = 30%
Riboflavin = 34%	Niacin = 28%	Vitamin C = 61%

SPAGHETTI WITH BEEF

LF, GF, SAFE (without onions, green peppers and tomatoes. Serve with cooked vegetables instead of salad), CHOL, DIAB, CH

Serves 1:

Brown 2 oz of ground beef (chuck or round). Add 2 cups of water, cover and simmer for one hour. Cool in refrigerator or freezer or add ice cubes. Skim off and discard the fat. Do not discard the juice. It contains many nutrients. Simmer it down without a cover. Add 3 ounces of tomato paste, 1 tbsp chopped onions, 2 tbsp chopped green peppers, one chopped garlic clove, 2 tsp dry basil, 1/4 tsp salt. Simmer for 1/2 hour and serve over spaghetti. Sprinkle with parmesan cheese. Serve with Italian bread, salad and fruit.

Nutrition Information for One Serving

Calories: 432
Protein = 26 gms   **Fat= 2 gms**   **Carbs = 23 gms**

Percent of the Recommended Dietary Allowances for the following leader nutrients:

Sodium = 28%	Potassium = 29%	Calcium = 10%
Iron = 40%	Vitamin A = 73%	Thiamin = 20%
Riboflavin = 14%	Niacin = 34%	Vitamin C = 88%

CHICKEN OR SHRIMP TETRAZZINI

LG, GF (substitute rice noodles for wheat noodles), SAFE (without onion and nutmeg. Serve with cooked vegetables instead of salad), CHOL, DIAB, PUL, CH

Serves 6:

On high heat cook enough chicken tenders to make 2 cups of cubed chicken for 8 minutes. Substitute shrimp but only cook for 3 minutes. Begin boiling with only 1/2 cup water. Add ice cubes when water starts to boil. Cool in refrigerator.

Sauce: Sauté in 2 tbsp butter, 1 cup fresh sliced mushrooms and 1 small chopped onion. Set aside.

In a large pan, stir until smooth 1/2 cup flour with 1/2 cup chicken broth. Add 1 cup chicken broth, 3/4 cup light cream, 1/2 cup milk, and 1/2 cup vermouth or dry white wine. Cook over medium heat and stir until smooth and bubbly. Add 1/2 tsp salt, 1/2 tsp nutmeg, and 2 tsp lemon juice. Remove from heat.

Take out 1/2 cup of sauce and stir into 2 beaten egg yolks. Stir as you add to the sauce. Combine the mushrooms, chicken and sauce.

In the meantime, cook 8 ounces of spaghetti in water. Drain. Add sauce to hot spaghetti and pour into a casserole. Sprinkle with 1/4 cup parmesan cheese. Bake 350° for one hour covered. Serve with rolls, salad and fruit.

Nutrition Information for One Serving. Serving size: 2 Cups.

Calories: 408

Protein= 23.4 gms	**Fat = 14.4 gms**	**Carbs = 44.5 gms**

Percent of the Recommended Dietary Allowances for the following leader nutrients:

Sodium = 24%	**Potassium = 11%**	**Calcium = 13%**
Iron = 16%	**Vitamin A = 11%**	**Thiamin = 27%**
Riboflavin = 30%	**Niacin = 55%**	**Vitamin C = 5%**

HAWAIIAN CHICKEN SALAD

LG, GF, SAFE (substitute sour cream for mayonnaise. Eliminate onion and curry powder. Eliminate cinnamon from cranberry bread recipe), CHOL, DIAB, PUL, CH

Serves 4:

Cook enough chicken tenders to make 1 1/2 cups of cubed chicken. Cool in refrigerator.

Boil 3/4 cup water and 1/2 tsp salt. Add 2/3 cup precooked instant rice. Remove from heat. Let stand covered for 13 minutes and uncovered for one hour. Refrigerate.

In a bowl combine 1 cup mayonnaise, 1 tsp lemon juice, 1 tsp grated onion, 1/2 tsp curry powder, 1/2 tsp salt, 1/8 tsp pepper, 1 cup chopped celery, 1/2 c shredded coconut, 1 cup unsweetened pineapple tidbits, 2 cups cold chicken. Fold in cold rice. Serve with cranberry bread, milk and fruit.

Nutrition Information for One Serving. Serving size: 1 1/3 Cups.

Calories: 380

Protein = 20 gms	Fat = 15.4 gms	Carbs = 46.4 gms

Percent of the Recommended Dietary Allowances for the following leader nutrients:

Sodium = 48%	Potassium = 15%	Calcium = 11%
Iron = 16%	Vitamin A = 11%	Thiamin = 28%
Riboflavin = 16%	Niacin = 46%	Vitamin C = 50%

POACHED CHICKEN BREASTS

LF, GF, SAFE, CHOL, DIAB, PUL, CH

Serves 4:

Poach 2 chicken breasts in 1 cup of chicken broth for 20 minutes.

Combine in a baking dish 1/2 cup plain skim milk yogurt with 1 tsp sesame oil or melted butter and 1 chopped anchovy filet. Add chicken breasts. Bake covered at 325° for 20 minutes. Serve with rice, bread, cooked vegetables and fruit.

Nutrition Information for One Serving. Serving size: 1/2 Chicken breast.

Calories: 176

Protein = 20 gms	Fat = 6.3 gms	Carbs = 8.7 gms

Percent of the Recommended Dietary Allowances for the following leader nutrients:

Sodium = 4 %	Potassium = 10%	Calcium = 29%
Iron = 4 %	Vitamin A = 4%	Thiamin = 8%
Riboflavin = 2.5%	Niacin = 37%	Vitamin C = 0%

Starches:

RAISIN BRAN MUFFINS WITH REDUCED SUGAR AND FAT

LF, GF, (Substitute Rice Flour for wheat flour), CHOL, DIAB, PUL, CH

Makes 56 Muffins but make as few as you want:

The dough can be stored in the refrigerator for 2 weeks.

Beat 4 eggs. Beat in 1/4 c sugar and 1/4 c oil or melted butter.

Mix together and add:

5 c Whole wheat flour

5 tsp Baking soda

1 pkg 15 oz Raisin Bran Cereal

2 cup All Bran

1 cup Unsweetened applesauce or apple juice concentrate.

1 qt Buttermilk

Spoon into baking cups and allow to stand for 20 minutes to allow the buttermilk to act.

Bake at 350° for 25 to 30 minutes

Nutrition Information for One Serving. Serving size: 1 Muffin.

Calories: 84

Protein = 3 gms	**Fat = 0.9 gms**	**Carbs = 18.4 gms**

Percent of the Recommended Dietary Allowances for the following leader nutrients:

Sodium = 7%	**Potassium = 3%**	**Calcium = 4%**
Iron = 25%	**Vitamin A = 8%**	**Thiamin = 19%**
Riboflavin = 16%	**Niacin = 13%**	**Vitamin C = 1%**

CRANBERRY BREAD

LF, GF, SAFE,(without cinnamon), CHOL, DIAB, PUL, CH

Makes 12 servings:

In large bowl combine 2 cups of whole wheat flour, 1 1/2 tsp of baking powder, 1/2 tsp baking soda, 1/2 tsp salt, 1/2 tsp cinnamon. Set aside. In another bowl mix 3/4 cup unsweetened applesauce, 1 beaten egg, 1 tbsp melted butter, 2 tsp vanilla extract. Pour liquid ingredients into dry ingredients. Add 1 1/2 cups of washed whole cranberries and mix well. Pour into greased loaf pan and bake at 350° for 45 minutes or until done. Allow to cool before cutting.

Nutrition Information for One Serving. Serving size: 1 Slice.

Calories: 84

Protein = 3 gms	**Fat = 0.9 gms**	**Carbs = 18.4 gms**

Percent of the Recommended Dietary Allowances for the following leader nutrients:

Sodium = 7%	**Potassium = 3%**	**Calcium = 4%**
Iron = 25%	**Vitamin A = 8%**	**Thiamin = 19%**
Riboflavin = 16%	**Niacin = 13%**	**Vitamin C = 1%**

BROWN RICE

LF, GF, SAFE, (without onions, green peppers and tomatoes or tomato juice), CHOL, DIAB, PUL, CH

Makes 5 cups with the added vegetables.

Heat add 4 cups of liquid (broth, tomato juice or water) in a covered pan.

Spread one cup of brown rice on cookie sheet. Toast under the broiler until brown (Stir often to prevent scorching).

Add rice to boiling liquid. Reduce heat to medium. Cover and simmer for 40 minutes.

In the meantime, simmer in broth or sauté in 1 tsp butter, 2 chopped onions and one chopped green pepper. Other vegetables such as tomatoes, peas, celery, mushrooms can be added.

Stir cooked vegetables into the cooked rice. Add salt if needed.

Nutrition Information for One Serving. Serving size: 3/4 Cup.

Protein = gms	**Fat = gms**	**Carbs = gms**

Percent of the Recommended Dietary Allowances for the following leader nutrients:

Sodium = 7%	**Potassium = 3%**	**Calcium = 4%**
Iron = 25%	**Vitamin A = 8%**	**Thiamin = 19%**
Riboflavin = 16%	**Niacin = 13%**	**Vitamin C = 1%**

Vegetables and Fruits:

CREAM DRESSING FOR FRUIT SALAD

LF, GF, SAFE (without cinnamon), PUL, CH

Makes 12 tbsp:

Mix 1 c sour cream with 1/4 c of undiluted frozen apple juice and 1 tbsp cinnamon or 1 tsp vanilla or almond extract.

Nutrition Information for One Serving. Serving size: 1 tbsp

Calories: 102
Protein = 1 gm	**Fat = 6 gms**	**Carbs = 11.1 gms**

Percent of the Recommended Dietary Allowances for the following leader nutrients:

Sodium = 1%	**Potassium = 3%**	**Calcium = 5%**
Iron = trace	**Vitamin A = 5%**	**Thiamin = Trace**
Riboflavin = trace	**Niacin = trace**	**Vitamin C = 0**

YOGURT DRESSING FOR FRUIT SALAD

LF, GF, CHOL, DIAB

Mix 1 cup skim milk yogurt with 1/4 cup of undiluted frozen apple juice and 1 tbsp cinnamon or 1 tsp vanilla or almond extract.

Nutrition Information for One Serving. Serving size: 1 tbsp

Calories: 52
Protein = 3.4 gm	**Fat = .1 gm**	**Carbs = 9.4 gms**

Percent of the Recommended Dietary Allowances for the following leader nutrients:

Sodium = 3%	**Potassium = 4%**	**Calcium = 15%**
Iron = 2%	**Vitamin A = trace**	**Thiamin = trace**
Riboflavin = trace	**Niacin = trace**	**Vitamin C = 0**

DRESSING WITHOUT OIL FOR VEGETABLE SALAD

LF, GF, SAFE (without lemon juice), CHOL, DIAB, CH

Makes 17 tbsp of dressing.

Shake together 1 cup buttermilk with 2 tsp lemon juice, 1/2 tsp dry basil, 1/2 tsp dry dill weed, 1/2 tsp of garlic powder, 1/2 tsp dried parsley, and 1/2 tsp salt.

Nutrition Information for One Serving: Serving size: 1 tbsp

Calories: 7
Protein = .5 gms	**Fat = .2 gms**	**Carbs = .9 gms**

Percent of the Recommended Dietary Allowances for the following leader nutrients:

Sodium = 3%	**Potassium = 1%**	**Calcium = 2%**
Iron = trace	**Vitamin A = 3%**	**Thiamin = trace**
Riboflavin = trace	**Niacin = trace**	**Vitamin C = 0**

Desserts:

SUGARLESS FROZEN STRAWBERRY CREAM

GF, SAFE (cook fruits for 2 minutes in microwave), PUL, CH

Make 4 servings:

Blend 2 cups washed strawberries and 2 bananas with 6 tbsp of heavy cream, 1 tsp vanilla extract and 1 cup whole milk. Freeze for 1 hour and then beat. Freeze again or serve.

Nutrition Information for One Serving. Serving size: 3/4 Cup

Calories: 195
Protein = 4.4 gms   **Fat = 10 gms**   **Carbs = 23.9 gms**

Percent of the Recommended Dietary Allowances for the following leader nutrients:

Sodium = 2%	**Potassium = 13%**	**Calcium = 15%**
Iron = 4%	**Vitamin A = 15%**	**Thiamin = 7%**
Riboflavin = 17%	**Niacin = 6%**	**Vitamin C = 85%**

YOGURT FRUIT SMOOTHIE

LF, GF, SAFE, (cook fruits in microwave for 2 minutes), CHOL, DIAB

Makes 4 servings:

In a blender blend 2 cups washed strawberries and 2 bananas with 1 1/4 cups skim milk yogurt, 2 tbsp of heavy cream and 1 tsp vanilla extract. Freeze for 1 hour then beat and freeze again or serve.

Nutrition Information for One Serving. Serving size: 3/4 Cup

Calories: 147
Protein = 8 gms   **Fat = .7 gms**   **Carbs = 28.6 gms**

Percent of the Recommended Dietary Allowances for the following leader nutrients:

Sodium = 4%	**Potassium = 17%**	**Calcium = 31%**
Iron = 5%	**Vitamin A = 4%**	**Thiamin = 9%**
Riboflavin = 25%	**Niacin = 6%**	**Vitamin C = 85%**

SUGARLESS RICE OR CORN MEAL PUDDING

LF, GF, SAFE, PUL, CH

Makes 4 servings:

Mix 1/2 cup of uncooked rice or corn meal with 2 tbsp light coffee cream, 1/2 cup whole milk, 1 beaten egg, 3 tsp melted butter, 1 tsp vanilla extract, and 1/2 cup of unsweetened crushed pineapple. Bake 325° for 30 minutes in a shallow 8x8 pan set in another pan with 1 inch of water.

Nutrition Information for One Serving: Serving size: 3/4 Cup

Calories: 178
Protein = 4.3 gms   Fat = 7 gms   Carbs = 23.9 gms

Percent of the Recommended Dietary Allowances for the following leader nutrients:

Sodium = 13%   Potassium = 2%   Calcium = 7%
Iron = 5%   Vitamin A = 7%   Thiamin = 8%
Riboflavin = 11%   Niacin = 5%   Vitamin C = 7%

SUGARLESS LOW FAT RICE OR CORN MEAL PUDDING

LF, GF, SAFE, CHOL, DIAB

Makes 4 servings:

Mix 1/2 cup of uncooked rice or corn meal, 1/2 cup skim milk, 1 beaten egg, 1 tsp melted butter, 1/2 tsp vanilla extract, and 1/2 cup of unsweetened crushed pineapple. Bake 325° for 25 minutes in a shallow 8x8 pan.

Nutrition Information for One Serving. Serving size: 3/4 Cup

Calories: 154
Protein = 4.1 gms   Fat = 4.5 gms   Carbs = 23.7 gms

Percent of the Recommended Dietary Allowances for the following leader nutrients:

Sodium = 13%   Potassium = 3%   Calcium = 7%
Iron = 6%   Vitamin A = 7%   Thiamin = 10%
Riboflavin = 10%   Niacin = 5%   Vitamin C = 7%

FANCY SUGARLESS INDIAN PUDDING

LF, GF, SAFE, CHOL, DIAB, CH, PUL (if served with cream).

Makes 4 servings:

Mix 2 cups of cooked grits or corn meal with 1 cup unsweetened crushed pineapple, 1 tsp vanilla extract, 1/2 tsp salt, 1 banana, 2 tbsp grated coconut. Bake at 350° for 20 minutes in a 8x8 pan.

Nutrition Information for One Serving: Serving size: 3/4 Cup

Calories: 145
Protein = 2.3 gms   Fat = 1 gms   Carbs = 32.4 gms

Percent of the Recommended Dietary Allowances for the following leader nutrients:

Sodium = 13%   Potassium = 5%   Calcium = 1%
Iron = 3%   Vitamin A = 5%   Thiamin = 8%
Riboflavin = 5%   Niacin = 5%   Vitamin C = 12%

SUGARLESS APPLE CRISP

LF, GF, SAFE, CHOL, DIAB, CH, PUL (if served with cream).

Makes 6 servings:

Mix 4 chopped and peeled apples with 1 cup unsweetened pineapple juice, 1/4 cup cornstarch, 1/2 tsp vanilla extract, and 1/2 cup of shredded coconut. Bake at 350° in a round cake pan for 25 minutes.

Nutrition Information for One Serving: Serving size: 3/4 Cup

Calories: 132

Protein = 1 gm	Fat = 2.7 gms	Carbs = 27.2 gms

Percent of the Recommended Dietary Allowances for the following leader nutrients:

Sodium = 0%	Potassium = 5%	Calcium = 2%
Iron = 2%	Vitamin A = 3%	Thiamin = 5%
Riboflavin = 2%	Niacin = 2%	Vitamin C = 15%

FRESH FRUIT MIX

LF, GF, CHOL, DIAB, CH, PUL (if served with cream).

Makes 20 servings

Cut up 10 cups of fresh fruit: bananas, apples, pears, oranges, melon, grapes, peaches, etc. In a double boiler, mix 4 tbsp of cornstarch, 1/2 cup of orange juice, 1/2 cup of unsweetened pineapple juice and 1 tbsp of lemon juice. Over simmering water, stir mix until clear. Immediately pour over fruit and toss with two forks so that all fruit is coated. Leave out to cool. Cover and refrigerate. Fruit will remain fresh looking without browning for 3 days.

Nutrition Information for One Serving: Serving size: 1/2 Cup

Calories: 52

Protein = .68 gms	Fat = .27 gms	Carbs = 12.9 gms

Percent of the Recommended Dietary Allowances for the following leader nutrients:

Sodium = 0%	Potassium = 4%	Calcium = 1%
Iron = trace	Vitamin A = 7%	Thiamin = trace
Riboflavin = trace	Niacin = trace	Vitamin C = 23%

UPSIDE DOWN FRUIT CAKE

LF, GF, SAFE, CHOL, DIAB, CH, PUL (if served with cream).

Makes 12 servings:

Peel and cut up 6 pounds of peaches or apples (pitted cherries or blueberries (not for safe diet) can be used too). Set aside.

Mix together 1 cup flour, 1/2 tsp salt, 3 tsp baking powder, 1/4 cup milk, 1 egg, 1/4 cup unsweetened frozen undiluted apple juice, 1 tsp sugar. Set aside. In a 8x12 pan melt 4 tbsp. butter in a 425° oven. While sizzling pour in the batter. Sprinkle peach slices over the batter. Bake 425° for 20 minutes.

Nutrition Information for One Serving: Serving size: 1 Slice
Calories: 108

| Protein = 3.3 gms | Fat = 2.9 gms | Carbs = 18.3 gms |

Percent of the Recommended Dietary Allowances for the following leader nutrients:

Sodium = 7%	Potassium = 3%	Calcium = 3%
Iron = 7%	Vitamin A = 2%	Thiamin = 12%
Riboflavin = 3%	Niacin = 6%	Vitamin C = trace

FOOD AND NUTRITION BOARD, NATIONAL ACADEMY OF SCIENCES-NATIONAL RESEARCH COUNCIL

RECOMMENDED DIETARY ALLOWANCES, revised, 1989*

	lbs	inches	K cal	protein (gms)	vit. A (iu)	vit. D (iu)	vit. E (iu)	vit. K (ug)	vit. C (mg)	vit. B2 (mg)	riboflavin (mg)	niacin (mg)	vit. B6 (mg)	folic acid (mg)	vit. B12 (ug)	calc (mg)	phos (mg)	mag (mg)	iron (mg)	zinc (mg)
Infants																				
0.0-0.5	13	24	651	13	1875	300	30	5	30	0.3	0.4	5	0.3	0.025	0.03	400	300	40	6	5
0.5-1.0	20	28	851	14	1875	400	40	10	35	0.4	0.5	6	0.6	0.035	0.05	600	500	60	10	5
Children																				
1-3	29	35	1300	16	2000	400	60	15	40	0.7	0.8	9	1.0	0.051	0.07	800	800	80	10	10
4-6	44	44	1800	24	2500	400	70	20	45	0.9	1.1	12	1.1	0.075	1.1	800	800	120	10	10
7-10	62	52	2000	28	3500	400	70	30	45	1.0	1.2	13	1.4	0.101	1.4	800	800	170	10	10
Males																				
11-14	99	62	2500	45	5000	400	100	45	50	1.3	1.5	17	1.7	0.151	2.1	1200	1200	270	12	15
15-18	145	69	3000	59	5000	400	100	65	60	1.5	1.8	20	2.0	0.201	2.1	1200	1200	400	12	15
19-24	160	70	2900	58	5000	400	100	70	60	1.5	1.7	19	2.0	0.201	2.1	1200	1200	350	10	15
25-50	174	70	2900	63	5000	200	100	80	60	1.5	1.7	19	2.0	0.201	2.1	800	800	350	10	15
51+	170	68	2300	63	5000	200	100	80	60	1.2	1.4	15	2.0	0.201	2.1	800	800	350	10	15
Females																				
11-14	101	62	2200	46	4000	400	80	45	50	1.1	1.3	15	1.4	0.151	2.1	1200	1200	280	15	12
15-18	120	64	2200	44	4000	400	80	55	60	1.1	1.3	15	1.5	0.181	2.1	1200	1200	300	15	12
19-24	128	65	2200	46	4000	400	80	60	60	1.1	1.3	15	1.6	0.181	2.1	1200	1200	280	15	12
25-50	138	64	2200	50	4000	200	80	65	60	1.1	1.3	15	1.6	0.181	2.1	800	800	280	15	12
51+	143	63	1900	50	4000	200	80	65	60	1.0	1.2	13	1.6	0.181	2.1	800	800	280	10	12
Pregnant			300	60	4000	400	100	65	70	1.5	1.6	17	2.2	0.401	2.2	1200	1200	320	30	15
Lactating																				
1st 6 mo.			500	65	6500	400	120	65	95	1.6	1.8	20	2.1	0.281	2.6	1200	1200	355	15	19
2nd 6 mo.			500	62	6500	400	110	65	90	1.6	1.7	20	2.1	0.261	2.6	1200	1200	340	15	16

Source: Recommended Dietary Allowances, 10th Edition. ©1989 by the National Academy of Sciences, National Academy Press, Washington, D.C.

*Reprinted with permission from the National Academy of Sciences, Washington, D.C.

Date	Time	Food Consumed	Beverage Consumed	Medication	Vitamin Supplement	Sub. Contact w/Skin	Substance Inhaled	Reaction

Diary to determine substance which may cause a reaction

Meal	Date/Time	Meat Protein Zinc Phosphorus Iron	Starch Carbohydrates Vitamin D Fiber	Fat	Vegetables Fiber Potassium Magnesium Vitamins A, B, C B6	Fruit Potassium Magnesium Vitamins A, B	Milk Protein Calcium Riboflavin Phosphorus	Non-Food	Feelings	Exercise Minutes
Breakfast										
Lunch										
Dinner										
Snack										
Breakfast										
Lunch										
Dinner										

Meal	Date/Time	Meat Protein Zinc Phosphorus Iron	Starch Carbohydrates Vitamin D Fiber	Fat	Vegetables Fiber Potassium Magnesium Vitamins A, B, C B6	Fruit Potassium Magnesium Vitamins A, B	Milk Protein Calcium Riboflavin Phosphorus		Non-Food	Feelings		Exercise Minutes
Snack												
Breakfast												
Lunch												
Dinner												
Snack												

Daily Diary

The Food Guide Pyramid
A Guide to Daily Food Choices

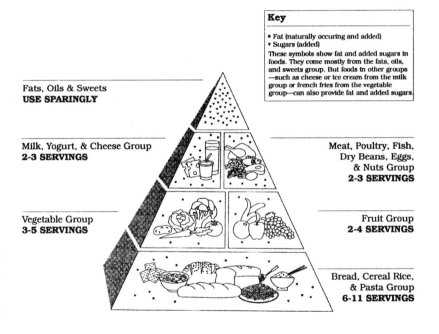

Key

• Fat (naturally occuring and added)
▼ Sugars (added)

These symbols show fat and added sugars in foods. They come mostly from the fats, oils, and sweets group. But foods in other groups —such as cheese or ice cream from the milk group or french fries from the vegetable group—can also provide fat and added sugars.

Fats, Oils & Sweets
USE SPARINGLY

Milk, Yogurt, & Cheese Group
2-3 SERVINGS

Meat, Poultry, Fish, Dry Beans, Eggs, & Nuts Group
2-3 SERVINGS

Vegetable Group
3-5 SERVINGS

Fruit Group
2-4 SERVINGS

Bread, Cereal Rice, & Pasta Group
6-11 SERVINGS

BIBLIOGRAPHY

Resources Used:

Books

Allen, A.M., *Food Medication Interactions*, 7th ed., 1991:159.

Anderson, L, Dibble, M. Turkki, P., Mitchell, H., & Rynbergen, H., *Nutrition in Health & Disease*, 17th ed., Philadelphia: J.B. Lippincott Company, 1982.

Bailey, Covert., *Fit or Fat*, Boston: Houghton Mifflin, 1978.

Benner, J., *Smoking Cigarettes*, Santa Barbara, CA: Joelle Publishing, 1987:53-55.

Berkow, R. ed., *The Merck Manual of Diagnosis & Therapy*, 15 ed. Rahway, NJ: Merck & Co. Inc., 1987:792.

Behrman, R.A. Kliegman, R.M., Nelson, W.E., & Vaughan III, V.C., *Nelson's Textbook of Pediatrics*, 14th ed., Philadelphia: W.B. Saunders, 1992:107.

Behrman, R.E. Kliegman, R.M. & Arvin, A.M., ed., *Nelson's Textbook of Pediatrics*, 15th ed., 1996:1567-1573.

Biochemistry of Vitamin A, Boca Raton, FL: CRC Press, 1989.

Biological Therapies in Psychiatry, Littleton, MA: PSG-Wright, Inc., March, 1981.

Brazelton, Berry, M.D., *Touchpoint*, Reading, Ma: Addison-Wesley Publishing, 1992.

Christian, Janet L. & Greger, Janet L., *Nutrition for Living*, Third ed, Redwood City, CA: Benjamin/Cummings Publishing Company, 1991.

Cooper, Kenneth., *Controlling Cholestero: Dr. Kenneth Cooper's Preventative Medicine Program*, Toronto, NY: Bantam Books, 1988.

Cooper, K., *Preventing Osteoporosis*, New York: Bantam Books, 1989:7.

Diehl, H.S., *Tobacco & Your Health-The Smoking Controversy*, 1969: 82.

Dudek, S.G., *Nutrition Handbook for Nursing Practice*, Philadelphia: Lippincott, 1987:564, 59, 56, 250 & 36-39.

Encyclopedia Britannica. Macropaedia, University of Chicago, Vol. 15:596.

Ferguson, T., *The Smoker's Book of Health*, Los Angeles: Putnam & Sons, 1987:36.

Goldbeck, Nikki, & Goldbeck, David., *The Goldbecks' Guide to Good Food*, New York: New American Library, 1987:180.

Guthrie, Helen A., *Introductory Nutrition*, 7th ed, Dubuque, IA: Times Mirror/Mosby College Publishing, 1989.

Hamilton, E.M.N., Whitney, E.N., & Sizer, F.S., *Nutrition Concepts & Controversies* 5th ed. St. Paul, MN: West Pub. 1991.

Hausman, Patricia., *The Calcium Bible. How to Have Better Bones All Your Life*, New York: Rawson Associates,1985:117-130.

Heany, R.P. & Barger, J.M., *Calcium & Common Sense*, New York: Doubleday, 1988:10-11.

Jagerstad, M., *The Role of Calcium in Biological Systems*, Vol 3, Boca Raton, Fl: CRC Press Inc., 1982:45-54.

Kahn, R.C. & Weir, G.C., *Joslin's Diabetes Mellitus*, Lea & Febiger, 1994:976-999, 196, 889 & 742-744.

Katch, F.I., & V.L., & McArdle, W.D., *Exercise Physiology*, Lea & Febiger, 1981:372-389.

Leslie, Stephen W., *Impotence: Current Diagnosis & Treatment*, Geddings D. Osborn Sr. Foundation, May 1990:2.

Long, J.W., *The Essential Guide to Prescription Drugs*, New York: Harper & Row, 1985.

Madar, Sylvia S., *Biology*, 3rd ed., Wm. C. Brown Pub, 1990:520.

Martens, R.A. & Martens, S., *The Milk Sugar Dilemma: Living with Lactose Intolerance*, 2nd ed., Santa Fe, NM: Health Press, 1988.

McIlwain, H.H.; Bruce, D.F.; Silverfield, J.C. & Burnette, M.C., *Osteoporosis*, John Wiley & Sons, Inc., 1988:11-36.

McWilliams, M., *Nutrition for the Growing Years*, 3rd ed., John Wiley & Sons, 1980.

The Medical Letter Handbook of Non-Prescription Drugs, The Medical Letter, Inc., 1993.

Neiman, D.E., Butterworth, D.E., & Nieman, C.E., *Nutrition*, First ed., Wm.C. Brown, 1990.

Ochsner, A., *Smoking Your Choice Between Life & Death*, New York: Simon & Schuster, 1970:110.

Paige, D.M., & Bayless, T.M. eds., *Lactose Digestion. Clinical & Nutritional Implications*, Baltimore: Johns Hopkins U. Press, 1981.

Perkins, J.E., *Food Allergies & Adverse Reactions*, Gaithersburg, MD: Aspen Pub., 1990: 210-219.

Pronsky, Zaneta M., *Food Medication Interactions*, 8th ed, 1993:72; 126.

Remington, Dennis W., & Higa, B.W., *The Bitter Truth About Artificial Sweeteners*, Vitality House International, 1987:27-36.

Rossman, Isadore, ed., *Clinical Geriatrics*, Philadelphia: J.D. Lippincott Co. 1971:391-403.

Robinson, Corinne, & Lawlar, Marilyn., *Normal & Therapeutic Nutrition*, Indianapolis: MacMillan Pub.

Roe, Daphne., *Handbook on Drug & Nutrient Interactions*, 4th ed., Chicago: American Dietetic Association, 1989.

Scrimshaw, N.S., & Young, V.R., *The Requirements of Human Nutrition,* Lea & Febiger, 1972:117.

Shils, Maurice E., & Young, Vernon R., *Modern Nutrition in Health & Disease,* 7th ed., Lea & Febiger, 1988.

Shivichan, H., *Clinical Advances: Pediatric Clinics of North America,* Philadelphia: Saunders, May 1954:389-403.

Schwartz, George R., *In Bad Taste,* Baltimore: Health Press, 1988.

The Human Body, Illustration, New York: Torstar Books, 1988.

Urgang, Laurence Associates, Ltd., *Dictionary of Medical Practice,* New York: Bantam Books, 1982:236.

Wardlaw, G.M., Insel, P.M., & Seyler, M. F., *Contemporary Nutrition,* Mosby Yearbook, 1992.

Winick, Myron, ed., *Nutrition & Aging,* New York: John Wiley Pub., 1976:131-144.

Whitney, E.R. & Rolfes, S.R., *Understanding Nutrition,* 6th ed., St. Paul, MN: West Pub., 1993.

Whitney, E.N., & Cataldo, C.B., *Understanding Normal & Clinical Nutrition,* St. Paul, MN: West Pub, 1983.

Wurtman, Richard, J., & Ritter-Walker, Eva., *Dietary Phenylalanine & Brain Functioning,* Cambridge, MA: Birkhauser, 1988:391.

Winick, Myron. ed., *Nutrition & Exercise,* New York: John Wiley & Sons, 1991:183-201.

Zeman, Frances J. & Ney, Denise M., *Applications of Clinical Nutrition,* Englewood Cliffs, NJ: Prentice Hall, 1988:223.

Periodicals.

Advances in Internal Medicine, (1990) Vol. 35:93.

American Journal of Cardiology, (1992) Vol. 69:1643-1644 & (1994) Vol. 73: 1227-1229.

American Journal of Clinical, (1982) Vol. 36:617-625 & 776; (1985) Vol. 42: 289-295 & 1994; (1991) Vol. 53:1104-1111; Vol. 54:157-163 & 197, (1992) Vol. 55:1060-1070; (1994) Vol. 60:735-738.

American Journal of the Disabled Child (1974) 537-540 & 890-891.

American Journal of Gastroenterology (1988) Vol. 83:538-540.

American Journal of Medicine (1987) Vol. 256:2394-2395; (1991) Vol. 265:1133-1138; (1993) Vol. 273:69.

The American Journal of Obstetrics & Gynecology (1977) March: 599-602.

Annals of Allergy, Asthma, & Immunology (1985) Vol. 54:538-540.

Journal of American College of Nutrition (1992) Vol. 11:567-783.

American Journal of Public Health (1990) Vol. 80:1323-1329.

Annals of Internal Medicine (1991) Vol. 114:128-132.

Annual Review of Medicine (1989) Vol. 40:251.

Archives of Internal Medicine (1983) Vol. 143. 1678-1682; (1992) Vol. 152:775-780.

Bone & Mineral Research (1988) Vol. 85:17-20.

The British Medical Journal (1979) Sept. 764-765; (1991) Vol. 303:17-20.

Canadian Family Physician (1991) Vol. 37:673-677.

Chest (1984) Vol . 85:411-41.

The Child's Doctor (1993) Fall: 4-8.

Circulation (1981) Vol. 63:1199A; (1992) Vol. 86:803-811 & 1046-1060; Vol. 88: 6.

Clinical Chemistry (1979) Vol. 25:523-525.

Clinical Pharmacy (1983) Vol. 3:152-162.

Consultant (1976) Nov. 59-69.

Contemporary Nutrition (1978) Vol. 3 # 3; (1991) Vol. 16 #3.

Contemporary Pediatrics (1995) Vol. 11:19-34 & 119.

Currents in Affective Illness (1986) Vol. 5 #2.

Diabetes (1952) Vol. 1:490-491; (1989) Vol. 38:141.

Diabetes Care (1992) Vol. 15:1361-1368.

Digestive Diseases (1976) Vol. 21:946-952.

Drug Therapy (1989) pg. 14-23.

Pediatric Emergency Care (1995) Vol. 11:11-13.

European Journal of Clinical Nutrition (1993) Vol. 47:828-839.

Food Technology (1989) Vol. 43:46.

Geriatrics(1980) Feb: 95-102.

Hospital Practice (1977) March: 121-128; (1979) Feb: 61-69; (1990) July: 95-108 & Vol. 25:38; (1991) Feb: 31-39; (1992) July 15; (1993) April 30; (1994) May: 45-52.

Indiana Medicine (1984) June: 441-445 & 463-464.

Journal of the American Dietetic Association (1990) Vol. 92:89-91 & 942-948 & 1139-1142; (1991) Vol. 91:430-434 & 1556-1564; (1993) Vol. 93:(1994) Vol. 94:841-842 & 976-985 & 1259-1269; (1996) Vol. 96:172-174.

Journal of the American Medical Association (1984) Vol. 252:2173-2176; (1992) Vol. 267:100-101 & 3317-3329; (1994) Vol. 272:1335-1374.

Journal of Atherosclerosis Research (1969) Vol. 9:251.

Journal of Laboratory Clinical Medicine (1982) Vol. 99:46.

Journal of Clinical Investigation (1991) Vol. 87:591-596; (1992) Vol. 89:1161.

Journal of Nutrition (1991) Vol. 120:13-23; (1992) Vol. 122:1119-1126.

Journal of Nutrition Education (1994) Vol. 26:278-283.

Journal Orthopedic Restoration (1989) Vol. 7:91-99.

Journal of Parenteral & Enteral Nutrition (1994) Vol. 18:544-548.

Journal of Respiratory Diseases (1994) Vol. 15:612-618.

Lancet (1989) Vol. 1:589; (1993) Nov. 1181-1185; (1992) 727-728.

Magnesium Research (1990) Vol. 3:197-215.

Mayo Clinic Proceedings (1993) Vol. 68:356; (1994) Vol. 69:462-466.

Medical Clinics of America (1981) Vol. 65. #4.

The Medical Letter (1993) Vol. 35:898.

Medical Science Sports Exercise (1993) Vol. 25. Supp.

Medical Tribune (1975) May 21.

Medicine (1978) Vol. 128:13.

Metabolism (1979) Vol. 28:373-385.

Neuroscience & Behavioral Reviews (1984) Vol. 8:503-513.

New England Journal of Medicine (1983) Vol. 308:1450-1466, Vol. 309: 431-432; (1986) Vol. 314:1676-1686; (1988) Vol. 318:818; (1990) Vol. 323: 480-481 & Vol. 324:912-913; (1992) Vol. 316:589, (1993) Vol. 328:308-311 & 1444-1449.

New York State Journal of Medicine (1975) Vol. 75:326-336.

Nutrition Abstracts & Reviews (1977) Vol. 47:579-582.

Nutrition Reviews (1989) Vol. 47:65.

Nutrition Today (1979) Nov/Dec. 26-32; (1988) Sept/Oct. 22.

Office Nurse (1993) June. 8-13.

Pediatrics (1992) Vol. 189:221-228.

Pediatric Annals (1990) Vol. 19:229; (1992) Vol. 21:676-687.

Pediatric News (1988) Vol. 22: 40.

Physician & Sports Medicine (1979) Vol. 7:49-61; (1982) Vol. 10: 202; (1990) Vol. 18:139-140; (1991) Vol. 19:17; (1992) Vol. 20:17-18; (1993) Vol. 21:43-46; (1994) Vol. 22:63-66; (1995) Vol. 23:15-16.

Postgraduate Medicine (1979) Vol. 1:66.

Practical Gastroenterology (1977) Vol. 1.

Science (1990) Vol. 207.

Science News (1991) Vol. 23:358.

Scientific American (1987) July 16; (1989) Nov. 22-23.

Seminars in Oncology (1983) Vol. 10:273.

World Review of Nutrition & Diet (1987) Vol. 50. 92-121.

Your Patient & Fitness (1991) Vol. 3. #1.

Organizations & Pamphlets.

"About Anorexia Nervosa," 1986, Scripographic Booklet. Channing L. Bete Co. Inc., South Deerfield, MA, 1985.

American College of Sports Medicine, 311 West Michigan St., Indianapolis, IN 46202.

Affiliate, Cleveland Clinic CompreCare, Cleveland, OH 44195-5124, Vol. 11, #1, May/June, 1996.

American Heart Association, 7272 Geenville Ave., Dallas, TX 75431.

American Academy of Pediatrics, 141 Northwest Point Blvd., Elk Grove Village, IL 60007.

Nutrition Reports. 1985, 1986, & 1992.

American Lung Association, 1740 Broadway, New York, NY 10012-2614.

Communique. Coldwell Banker. Available from local Real Estate Offices. Consumer Reports on Health. Consumer Reports, Dept. GH, 101 Truman Ave., Yonkers, NY 10703.

Contemporary Nutrition. General Mills, Inc., Box 1112, Dept. #65, Minneapolis, MN 55440.

Egg Nutrition Center, 1819 H St. NW #520, Room 331E, Washington, DC 20006.

Current Health, 245 Long Hill Rd., Box 2791, Middletown, CT 96457.

Diabetes. American Diabetes Association, 1660 Duke St., Alexandria, VA 22314.

Dairy Council Digest & Nutrition News. National Dairy Council, 10255 W. Higgins Rd., Rosemont, IL 60018.

Diabetes in the News, 1560 N. Sandburg Terrace, Apt. 1402, Chicago, IL 60610.

Diabetes literature. Eli Lilly & Company, Lilly Corporate Center, Indianapolis, IN 46285.

Diabetes Literature. Joslin Diabetes Center, 1 Joslin Place, Boston, MA 02215.

Environmental Nutrition, 512 Riverside Dr., Bldg. 15 A, New York, NY 10224.

Food & Nutrition News. The National Livestock & Meat Board, 444 N. Michigan, Chicago, IL 60611.

Health Update. Porter-Starke Counseling Centers, Porter-Starke Hospital, Valpariso, IN 46383.

Heart to Heart. Cardiology Associates, 621 Memorial Dr., South Bend, IN 46601.

Inside Tract. Glaxo Institute for Digestive Health, P.O. Box, 899, West Caldwell, NJ 07007.

Lactose Content Medications. McNeil Consumer Products Company, Camp Hill Rd., Fort Washington, PA 19034.

Massachusetts General Hospital Newsletter, 32 Fruit St. Boston, MA 02114.

Mayo Clinic Health Letter & Mayo Clinic Bulletin. Mayo Medical Ventures, 200 First St. S.W., Rochester, MN 55905.

Med Facts. National Jewish Center for Immunology & Respiratory Medicine, 1400 Jackson Rd., Denver, CO 80206.

Metabolic Currents. Ross Laboratories, Columbus, OH 43216.

National Institute of Allergy & Infectious Diseases, 31 Center Dr., MSC-2520 #7A50, Bethesda, MD 20892.

National Osteoporosis Foundation, 2100 M. St., NW, Suite 602, Washington, DC 20037.

National Research Council, National Academy of Sciences, Wash. DC, 2101 Constitution Ave. NW, Washington, DC 20418. "The Role of Dietary Fat in Human Health" Publication # 474.

Products & Literature Regarding Phenylketonuria. Mead Johnson Products, 2400 W. Lloyd Expwy, Evansville, IN 47721.

Nutrition Analysis Program. Anjon Systems, Inc., P.O. Box 4278, South Bend, IN 46634.

Nutrition Action Health Letter, Center for Science in the Public Interest, 1875 Connecticut Ave. NW, Washington, DC 20009.

Pharmacy Review, PCS Clinical Management Services, Pub. 5701 Green Vallery Dr., Minneapolis, MN 55437.

Practitioner's Consult, McNeil Consumer Products Company, Camp Hill Rd., Fort Washington, PA 19034.

Medical Staff LINC, St. Joseph Hospital, 215 W. 4th St., Mishawaka, IN 46545.

Tufts Medical & Diet newsletter, 53 Park Place, New York, NY 10007.

"Understanding Food Allergy." American Academy of Allergy & Immunology, 611 E. Wells St., Milwaukee, WI 53202.

University of California Wellness Letter, Health Letter Associates, 622 Broadway, New York, NY 10012.

Government Bulletins:

U.S. Dept. of Health & Human Services, National Heart, Lung, & Blood Institute, National Cholesterol Education Program, 200 C St. SW, Washington, DC 20204.

"Report of the Expert Panel on Population Strategies for Blood Cholesterol Reduction," National Institutes of Health (NIH) publication # 90-3046, 1990.

"High Blood Cholesterol in Adults," Jan. 1989, "National Institute of Health Consensus Development Conference on Triglycerides, HDL, & Coronary Heart Disease," Feb. 26-28, 1992.

"Report of the Expert Panel on Blood Cholesterol Levels in Children & Adolescents." NIH Publication #91-2732, Sept, 1991.

"So You Have High Blood Cholesterol," pg. 5, NIH Publication # 89-2922, 1989.

Food & Drug Administration Medical Bulletin, 5600 Fishers Lane, Rockville, MD 20857.

U.S. Dept. of Agriculture, Food, Nutrition & Consumer Services, 14th & Independence Ave. SW, Room 240E, Washington, DC 20250. *Nutritive Values of Foods*, Home & Garden Bulletin, No. 72, 1986.

Lectures.

Castelli, A.K., Framingham Research Center. (Lecture at Memorial Hospital, South Bend, Indiana, Sept., 24, 1986).

Palumbo, P.J., Mayo Clinic, Scottsdale, AZ "New Approaches to the Treatment of NIDDM." Lecturer at Memorial Hospital, South Bend, IN. October 7, 1995.

Popular Press.

American Health (1991) July/Aug: 18; (1984) March/April.

Health (1970) Sept/Oct:10.

Self (1982) Dec: 32-36; (1984) June: 160-162 & Jan: 128-129.

New Choices (1993) Dec: 22-23.

Fortune (1995) Dec. 11, : 164-174.

Good Housekeeping (1987) Feb: 202-203.

Lear's (1990) Sept: 74.

McCalls (1991) Sept: 12; (1989) Oct: 149.

New Yorker (1993) Sept 20, : 64-72.

Parade (1992) Sept. 13, : 20-23.

Parents Magazine (1993) July: 46.

Prevention (1991) Vol. 43:10.

Reader's Digest (1994) April: 129.

Time (1995) June 26.

Working Woman (1992) Sept: 94-109.

Weight Watcher Magazine (1995) June 22.

Newspapers.

The Herald Palladium (1990) Oct. 21. 1B.

The Naples Daily News (1995) April 6; (1995) Jan. 3; (1996) March 10; (1992) Jan. 28. 2D.

New York Times (1993) Dec. 17. C1 & 8.

The South Bend Tribune (1990) Sept. 9; (1993) May 2:10; (1994) May 16:1; (1992) Oct. 7:A 2; (1988) Jan. 25 & Oct. 12; (1982) Sept, 28; (1985) Jan. 28.

USA Today (1994) May 16:1; (1994) July 26; (1991) March 7; (1994) July 19:6D; (1990) Dec. 5; (1996) April 14.

REFERENCES

1. Bailey, Covert, *Fit or Fat*, Houghton Mifflin, Pub. 1978

2. Katch, Frank I., and Victor L., and McArdle, William D., *Exercise Physiology*, Lea & Febiger, Pub. 1981:372-389.

3. Whitney, Eleanor, and Cataldo, Corinne, *Understanding Normal and Clinical Nutrition*, West Pub, 1983:834.

4. *Recommended Dietary Allowances*, 10 ed., 1989, National Academy of Sciences Press, Washington, D.C.

5. Shils, M.E., and Young, V.R., *Modern Nutrition in Health and Disease*, 7th Ed., Lea & Febiger, Pub., 1988:76.

6. "Inside Tract," Glaxo Institute for Digestive Health, P.O. Box, 899, West Caldwell, N.J., 07007-0899.

7. Citkova, Renata, Memorial University of Newfoundland, St. John's Newfoundland, Canada, in Communique, Coldwell Banker, "Breakfast More Important Than You Think."

8. Grundy, S.M., "Hydrogenated Vegetable Fats Shown to Increase Serum Cholesterol," in New England Journal of Medicine, 1990 Vol. 323:480-81.

9. Health Update, "Health and Fitness Briefs," pub. by Porter Starke Counseling Centers, May 1995.

10. Burros, Marian, "Seafood, Even Shrimp, Approved for those with High Cholesterol," in South Bend Tribune, Jan. 25, 1988.

11. *Affiliate*, Vol 11, #1, May/June, 1996, Cleveland Clinic CompreCare, Cleveland, Ohio, 44195-5124.

12. *Physician's Desk Reference*, 1996, Medical Economics Co, Montvale, N.J.

13. *Pediatric News*, Vol.22, No.5, May, 1988:40.

14. Committee on Nutrition, American Academy of Pediatrics, Sept. 5, 1986.

15. *Contemporary Pediatrics*, Vol 11, June, 1995:119.

16. Newman, T.B., in *Journal of the American Medical Association*, Vol. 267, 1992:100-101.

17. Brazelton, Berry, M.D., *Touchpoint*, Addison-Wesley Publishing, 1992.

18. Round table with Ryan, Allan J., Leon, A.L., Etzwiler,D.L., Costill, D.L. and Zinman, B., "Diabetes and Exercise," in *The Physician and Sportsmedicine*, Vol. 7, # 3, March 1979:49-61.

19. Kaplan, N.M., "Syndromes X: Two Too Many," in American Journal of Cardiology, Vol. 69, June 15, 1992:1643-1644.

20. Mazze, R.S., in Mayo Clinic Proc., April 1993, Vol 68:356.

21. Joslin, E.P., "Appollinaire Bouchardat," -1806-1886, in Diabetes, Vol. 1, 1952:490-491.

22. *Dictionary of Medical Practice*, Prepared by Laurence Urdang Associates, Ltd.,Bantam Books, 1982.

23. Hasling, D;, Sondergaard, Kl; Charles, P. and Mosekilde, L., "Calcium Metabolism in Postmenopausal Osteoporatic Women is Determined by Dietary Calcium and Coffee Intake," in Journal of Nutrition, Vol 122, May 1992:1119-1126.

24. Painter, Kim, USA Today, July 19, 1994:6D.

25. Talan, J. The Male Hormone is a Female Hormone Too, in American Health, July/Aug., 1991:18.

26. *Vital Signs: in Health*, Sept/Oct, 1970:10

27. Clark, Nancy, "Athletes with Amenorrhea: Nutrition to the Rescue" in Physician and SportsMedicine, Vol 21, #4, 1993:45-46.

28. Carter, Betsy, "Estrogen Therapy" in Working Woman, Sept. 1992:94-96.

29. "Osteoporosis" in Contemporary Nutrition, Gen. Mills Pub. Jan. 1985, Vol.10, #1.

30. Carter, Betsy, "Estrogen Therapy" in Working Woman, Sept. 1992:94-96.

31. Wallis, C., "The Estrogen Dilemna" in Time, June 26, 1995.

32. Heaney, R.P. and Recker, R.R., "Effects of Nitrogen, Phosphorus and Caffeine on Calcium Balance in Women," in J.Lab.Clin. Med., Vol 99, 1982:46.

33. Heaney, R.P. and Recker, R.R., "Effects of Nitrogen, Phosphorus and Caffeine on Calcium Balance in Women," in J.Lab.Clin. Med., Vol. 99, 1982:46.

34. Wysak, G.; Frisch, R..E.; Albright, T.E.; et al, "NonAlcoholic Carbonated Beverage Consumption and Bone Fractures Among Women Former College Athletes" in J. Ortho Res, Vol 7, #1, 1989:91-99.

35. Cooper, Kenneth, *Preventing Osteoporosis*, Bantam Books, Pub., 1989.

36. National Academy of Sciences, Washington, D.C., Food and Nutrition Board, Recommended Dietary Allowances, 1989.

37. Slesinski, M.J., Subar, A.F., and Kahle, L.L., "Trends in Use of Vitamin and Mineral Supplements in United States-1987-1992 The National Health Interview Survey," in J. Amer. Diet Assoc., Vol. 95, #8:921-923.

38. Leonard, G., New Choices, Dec.1993: Jan.1994:22-23.

39. Lindeman, A.K., "Eating for Endurance or Ultra Endurance," Physician and SportsMedicine, Vol.20, #3, March, 1992.

40. Levy, D., "More Fat in Diet a Boost for Athletes" in USA Today, April 14, 1996.

41. "Balancing Heat, Stress. Fluids and Electrolytes" in Physician and SportsMedicine, Aug. 1975:43-48.

ADA Report, "Position Of American Dietetic Association and The Canadian Dietetic Association: Nutrition and Physical Fitness and Athletic Performance for Adults" in J. Amer. Diet. Assoc., June 1993, Vol. 93, No. 6

American Heart Association, "1990 Heart and Stroke Facts" and "Heart and Stroke Facts: 1995 Statistical Supplement,"

Cancer Facts and Figures: 1995-Amer. Cancer Society, Revised January, 1995.

Rothkopf, M.M., Askanazi, J.,"Nutrition and Respiration," (Unpublished) Veterans Administration Medical Center, East Orange, J., and Department of Anesthiology, College of Physicians and Surgeons, Columbia University, New York, NY.

*Other references to specific items within the text may be obtained from the author

INDEX

Books by Starburst Publishers

Eat for the Health of It   —Erickson & Dempsey

A back-to-basics approach to eating and learning how to maintain and preserve your body: Tells why some people gain weight on six grams of fat. Tells how to improve your health with or without medicine. Gives 21 reasons why blood cholestral rises. Contains hundreds of anecdotes, meal plans, resources and recipes. **Eat for the Health of It** will have you eating towards a better life!

(trade paper) ISBN 0914984780   **$15.95**

The Crystal Clear Guide to Sight for Life   —Gayton & Ledford

Subtitled: *A Complete Manual of Eye Care for Those Over 40*. **The Crystal Clear Guide to Sight For Life** makes eye care easy-to-understand by giving clear knowledge of how the eye works with the most up-to-date information available from the experts. Contains more than 40 illustrations, a detailed index for cross-referencing, a concise glossary, and answers to often-asked questions.

(trade paper) ISBN 0914984683   **$15.95**

Migraine—Winning The Fight of Your Life   —Charles Theisler

This book describes the hurt, loneliness and agony that migraine sufferers experience and the difficulty they must live with. It explains the different types of migraines and their symptoms, as well as the related health hazards. Gives 200 ways to help fight off migraines, and shows how to experience fewer headaches, reduce their duration, and decrease the agony and pain involved.

(trade paper) ISBN 0914984632   **$10.95**

Health, Happiness & Hormones   —Arlene Swaney

Subtitled: *One Woman's Journey Toward Health After a Hysterectomy*. A frightening and candid look into one woman's struggle to find a cure for her medical condition. In 1990, when her story was first published in *Prevention* magazine, author Arlene Swaney received an overwhelming response from women who also were plagued by mysterious, but familiar, symptoms leading to continuous misdiagnoses. Starting with a hysterectomy Swaney details the years of lost health that followed as she searched for an accurate diagnosis. Her story is told with warmth and compassion.

(trade paper) ISBN 0914984721   **$9.95**

Stay Well Without Going Broke   —Gulling, Renner, & Vargas

Subtitled: *Winning the War Over Medical Bills*. Provides a blueprint for how health care consumers can take more responsibility for monitoring their own health and the cost of its care—a crucial cornerstone of the health care reform movement today. Contains inside information from doctors, pharmacists and hospital personnel on how to get cost-effective care without sacrificing quality. Offers legal strategies to protect your rights when illness is terminal.

(hardcover) ISBN 0914984527   **$22.95**

The Low-Fat Supermarket   —Judith & Scott Smith

Subtitled: *A Guide to Weight-Loss, Cholesterol Control and Good Nutrition for the Entire Family*. A comprehensive reference of over 4,500 brand name products that derive less than 30% of their calories from fat. Information provided includes total calories, fat, cholesterol and sodium content. Organized according to the sections of a supermarket. Your answer to a healthier you.

(trade paper) ISBN 0914984438   **$10.95**

Books by Starburst Publishers —cont'd

Dr. Kaplan's Lifestyle of the Fit & Famous —Eric Scott Kaplan

Subtitled: *A Wellness Approach to "Thinning and Winning."* A comprehensive guide to the formulas and principles of: FAT LOSS, EXERCISE, VITAMINS, NATURAL HEALTH, SUCCESS and HAPPINESS. More than a health book—it is a lifestyle based on the empirical formulas of healthy living. Dr. Kaplan's food-combining principles take into account all the major food sources (fats, proteins, carbohydrates, sugars, etc.) that when combined within the proper formula (e.g. proteins cannot be mixed with refined carbohydrates) will increase metabolism and decrease the waistline. This allows you to eat the foods you want, feel great, and eliminate craving and binging.

(hardcover) ISBN 091498456X **$21.95**

The World's Oldest Health Plan —Kathleen O'Bannon Baldinger

Subtitled: *Health, Nutrition and Healing from the Bible.* Offers a complete health plan for body, mind and spirit, just as Jesus did. It includes programs for diet, exercise and mental health. Contains foods and recipes to lower cholesterol and blood pressure, improve the immune system and other bodily functions, reduce stress, reduce or cure constipation, eliminate insomnia, reduce forgetfulness, confusion and anger, increase circulation and thinking ability, eliminate "yeast" problems, improve digestion, and much more.

(trade paper-opens flat) ISBN 0914984578 **$14.95**

Allergy Cooking With Ease —Nicolette M. Dumke

Subtitled: *The No Wheat, Milk, Eggs, Corn, Soy, Yeast, Sugar, Grain, and Gluten Cookbook.* A book designed to provide a wide variety of recipes to meet many different types of dietary and social needs and, whenever possible, save you time in food preparation. Includes: Recipes for those special foods that most food allergy patients think they will never eat again; Timesaving tricks; and Allergen Avoidance Index.

(trade paper-opens flat) ISBN 091498442X **$12.95**

Home Business Happiness —Cheri Fuller

Subtitled: *Secrets On Keeping The Family Ship Afloat From Entrepreneurs Who Made It.* More than 26 million people in the U.S. work at home businesses. **Home Business Happiness** is your network for success! In a reader-friendly style. Author Cheri Fuller offers valuable advice from some of the most inventive and pioneering entrepreneurs in the country. Some of the topics included are: Starting a Home Business, Time Management, and Avoiding Potential Pitfalls.

(trade paper) ISBN 0914984705 **$12.95**

God Is! —Mark R. Littleton

"Heart-Tugging" inspirational stories, quotes & illustrations that will leave a powerful mental and emotional impact on the reader. Short and easy-to-read sketches, embracing the attributes of God, will inspire your spirit and brighten your day. Topics include, *God Is Love, God Is Good, God Is Wise* and more.

(hardcover) ISBN 0914984926 **$14.95**

Books by Starburst Publishers—cont'd

Parenting With Respect and Peacefulness   —Louise A. Dietzel

Subtitled: *The Most Difficult Job in the World.* Parents who love and respect themselves parent with respect and peacefulness. Yet, parenting with respect is the most difficult job in the world. This book informs parents that respect and peace communicate love—creating an atmosphere for children to maximize their development as they feel loved, valued, and safe. Parents can learn authority and control by a common sense approach to day-to-day situations in parenting.

(trade paper) ISBN 0914984667   **$10.95**

Grapes of Righteousness   —Joseph H. Powell

Subtitled: *Spiritual Grafting Into the True Vine.* Dr. Powell uses an analogy that compares and contrasts our development into God's kingdom under His hands, to the cultivating and nurturing of a vineyard by a gardener. Possessing a Ph.D in Botany, the author uses his extensive study of grafting, pruning, nutrition, and dormancy to illustrate the basic Biblical principles necessary to spiritual birth and subsequent growth and maturity.

(trade paper) ISBN 0914984748   **$10.95**

From Grandma With Love   —Ann Tuites

Subtitled: *Thoughts for Her Children Everywhere.* People are taught all kinds of things from preschool to graduate school, but they are expected to know instinctively how to get along with their families. Harmony within the home is especially difficult when an aging relative is involved. The author presents personal anecdotes to encourage caregivers and those in need of care. Practical, emotional and spiritual support is given so that all generations can learn to live together in harmony.

(hardcover) ISBN 0914984616   **$14.95**

Lease–Purchase America!   —John Ross

A first-of-its-kind book that provides a simple "nuts and bolts" approach to acquiring real estate. Explains how the lease-purchase technique pioneered by John Ross can now be used in real estate to more easily buy and sell a home. Details the value of John's technique from the perspective of each participant in the real estate transaction. Illustrates how the reader can use lease-purchase successfully as a tool to achieve his or her real estate goals.

(trade paper) ISBN 0914984454   **$9.95**

Purchasing Information:

Listed books are available from your favorite Bookstore, either from current stock or special order. To assist bookstores in locating your selection be sure to give title, author, and 10 digit ISBN #. If unable to purchase from the bookstore you may order direct from STARBURST PUBLISHERS. When ordering, enclose full payment plus $3.00 for shipping and handling ($4.00 if Canada or overseas). Payment in US Funds only. Please allow two to three weeks minimum (longer overseas) for delivery. Make checks payable to and mail to STARBURST PUBLISHERS, P.O. Box 4123, LANCASTER, PA 17604. **Prices subject to change without notice.** Catalog available for a 9 x 12 self-addressed envelope with 4 first-class stamps.   2-97